Understanding ABGs & Lung Function Tests

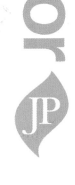

pocket tutor

Muhunthan Thillai MBBS MRCP
Specialty Trainee and Research Fellow
Imperial College London
London, UK

Keith Hattotuwa MBBS FRCP
Consultant Physician and Senior Lecturer
Department of Respiratory Medicine
Broomfield Hospital
Chelmsford, UK

JP
medical
publishers

© 2012 JP Medical Ltd.

Published by JP Medical Ltd, 83 Victoria Street, London, SW1H 0HW, UK

Tel: +44 (0)20 3170 8910 Fax: +44 (0)20 3008 6180

Email: info@jpmedpub.com Web: www.jpmedpub.com

The rights of Muhunthan Thillai and Keith Hattotuwa to be identified as the authors of this work have been asserted by them in accordance with the Copyright, Designs and Patents Act 1988.

All brand names and product names used in this book are trade names, service marks, trademarks or registered trademarks of their respective owners. The publisher is not associated with any product or vendor mentioned in this book.

Medical knowledge and practice change constantly. This book is designed to provide accurate, authoritative information about the subject matter in question. However, readers are advised to check the most current information available on procedures included or from the manufacturer of each product to be administered, to verify the recommended dose, formula, method and duration of administration, adverse effects and contraindications. It is the responsibility of the practitioner to take all appropriate safety precautions. Neither the publisher nor the authors assume any liability for any injury and/or damage to persons or property arising from or related to use of the material in this book.

This book is sold on the understanding that the publisher is not engaged in providing professional medical services. If such advice or services are required, the services of a competent medical professional should be sought.

Every effort has been made where necessary to contact holders of copyright to obtain permission to reproduce copyright material. If any have been inadvertently overlooked, the publisher will be pleased to make the necessary arrangements at the first opportunity.

ISBN: 978-1-907816-05-5

British Library Cataloguing in Publication Data
A catalogue record for this book is available from the British Library

Library of Congress Cataloging in Publication Data
A catalog record for this book is available from the Library of Congress

JP Medical Ltd is a subsidiary of Jaypee Brothers Medical Publishers (P) Ltd, New Delhi, India

Publisher:	Richard Furn
Development Editor:	Paul Mayhew
Editorial Assistant:	Katrina Rimmer
Design:	Designers Collective Ltd
Index:	Indexing Specialists (UK) Ltd

Typeset, printed and bound in India.

Foreword

More than 2,400 years ago, when Hippocrates was laying down the principles of medicine in the book of Prognostics he said: "It appears to me a most excellent thing for the physician to cultivate Prognosis; for by foreseeing and foretelling, in the presence of the sick, the present, the past, and the future… he will be the more readily believed to be acquainted with the circumstances of the sick". When faced with a patient with lung disease, the interpretation of physiological measures of pulmonary function is vital in modern prognostics.

The science behind physiological measurement of the severity of lung disease is relatively recent, mostly developed over the past 100 years. After much discussion and debate the clinical use of tests has now more or less reached a stable consensus. Although interpretation of commonly used tests is not technically very complex, many medical students and young doctors (and even some older doctors) struggle with how to best to interpret and use pulmonary test results.

These simple tests enormously enhance our ability to diagnose and stage disease, to decide on treatments and level of care. When assessing a patient we take a history, we perform a physical examination and we request tests. When the history and examination is in line with the test results we feel reassured and know how to proceed with confidence. When the test results are out of line, we need to work out why: the breathless patient with normal lung function is likely to have either an interesting and unexpected disease, or perhaps a complex psychosocial background that needs to be explored.

The interpretation of commonly performed pulmonary function tests is not hard; it just needs to be clearly explained. This book is just what the practising doctor needs to make sense of these tests and to use them to improve clinical care. Whether you want to be the next Hippocrates or just to get through the next ward round, you will learn a lot from reading it.

Peter JM Openshaw FRCP PhD FMedSci
Professor of Experimental Medicine
National Heart & Lung Institute
Imperial College London
London, United Kingdom

Preface

The spirometer was invented in 1842 by an English surgeon named Jonathan Hutchinson who noted that the air which was exhaled from a fully inflated lung was a powerful indicator of longevity. His basic spirometer measured the *capacity to live*, otherwise known as the vital capacity. The first accurate measurement of blood gases occurred at a similar time when, in 1837, a German physicist named Gustav Magnus experimented on 'commoners who for a small sum permitted themselves to be bled.'

Although technology has evolved since the first measurements of arterial blood gases (ABGs) and lung function more than 150 years ago, the basic approach to interpreting the results has remained largely constant. A clear understanding of these tests will allow you to rapidly assess critically unwell patients, plan for long-term management and assess a person's fitness prior to surgery.

In this book, we begin with an overview of respiratory anatomy, physiology and biochemistry. We describe key respiratory terminology and then provide a step-by-step guide to understanding the tests, defining normal results and interpreting key abnormalities. This background information (chapters 1–3) is then used to explain common systemic ABG and lung function abnormalities (chapters 4–8).

Disorders are illustrated by representative test results and brief accompanying text which clearly identifies the defining abnormalities. This book can serve as a handy companion for quick reference during teaching, as a revision tool before examinations and for daily use on the wards. We have tried to use as many real-life clinical scenarios as possible and hope that you can use this information as a guide to interpreting ABG and lung function results in your own daily clinical practice.

Muhunthan Thillai
Keith Hattotuwa
August 2011

Contents

Glossary

Respiratory variables

AT	anaerobic (or lactate) threshold
ERV	expiratory reserve volume
FEF	forced expiratory flow
$FEV_{0.75}$	forced expiratory volume in 0.75 second
FEV_1	forced expiratory volume in 1 second
F_iO_2	fraction of inspired oxygen
FRC	functional residual capacity
FVC	forced vital capacity
IC	inspiratory capacity
IRV	inspiratory reserve volume
MBC	maximum breathing capacity
MEP	maximum expiratory pressure
MIP	maximum inspiratory pressure
MMEF	maximal midexpiratory flow
MMV	maximum voluntary ventilation
MVV	maximum voluntary ventilation
P_aO_2 and P_aCO_2	partial pressures of oxygen and carbon dioxide in arterial blood
P_AO_2	partial pressure of oxygen within the alveoli
$P_{A-a}O_2$	alveolar–arterial oxygen gradient
P_B	barometric pressure
P_iO_2	partial pressure of inspired oxygen
PC_{20}	concentration of drug required to provoke a 20% reduction in FEV_1
PH_2O	pressure of water vapour in air
P_{DI}	transdiaphragmatic pressure
PEF	peak expiratory flow
PEFR	peak expiratory flow rate
PIFR	peak inspiratory flow rate
P_{Emax}	maximal expiratory pressure

P_{Imax}	maximal inspiratory pressure
$\dot{Q}_c$	overall perfusion of the pulmonary capillaries
$\dot{Q}_s/\dot{Q}_T$	Shunt component
R	respiratory quotient
RMV	resting minute ventilation
RR	respiratory rate
RV	residual volume
S_aO_2	saturation of haemoglobin with oxygen in arterial blood
SVC	slow vital capacity
TLC	total lung capacity
T_LCO	transfer factor of CO
$\dot{V}CO_2$	amount of CO_2 produced in the lungs per minute
$\dot{V}O_{2peak}$	rate of O_2 consumption at maximum attainable exercise
$\dot{V}_a$	ventilation of the alveoli
$\dot{V}/\dot{Q}$	ventilation–perfusion quotient
V_T	tidal volume
VC	vital capacity
WV	walking ventilation

Abbreviations

ABG	arterial blood gas
AHI	apnoea/hypopnoea index
ALS	amyotrophic lateral sclerosis
ARDS	acute respiratory distress syndrome
ASD	atrial septal defect
BOOP	bronchiolitis obliterans organising pneumonia
BPAP	bilevel positive airway pressure
COPD	chronic obstructive pulmonary disease
CO_2	carbon dioxide
CPAP	continuous positive airway pressure
CRP	C-reactive protein
CT	computed tomography
DKA	diabetic ketoacidosis
ECG	electrocardiogram
EEG	electroencephalogram

EMG	electromyogram
EOG	submental
HONK	hyperosmotic non-ketotic
LEMS	Lambert–Eaton myasthenic syndrome
LFT	Lung function test
MND	motor neuron disease
NREM	non-rapid eye movement
O_2	oxygen
OSAHS	obstructive sleep apnoea/hypopnoea syndrome
REM	rapid eye movement
WCC	white cell count

First principles

An understanding of lung function and gaseous exchange is essential to the practice of cardiorespiratory medicine and lung function tests (LFTs) and arterial blood gases (ABGs) are part of everyday clinical practice. The principal clinical uses of LFTs and ABGs are in:

- Diagnosing respiratory and cardiac disease
- Assessing the severity of both acute (e.g. chronic obstructive pulmonary disease or COPD) and acute-on-chronic (e.g. muscular dystrophy) disease
- Measuring the response to management, e.g. the efficacy of steroid inhalers in asthma
- Preoperative safety checks
- Postoperative and critical care monitoring

The assessment of lung function provides vital information, especially when the signs and symptoms of lung disease are subclinical. Respiratory function may be severely impaired and yet the lungs may appear normal on a chest radiograph. Conversely, gross radiological abnormalities may be associated with only mild impairment of physiological function.

A basic understanding of the theories behind these investigations, as well as the ability to interpret abnormalities, is vital when diagnosing disorders as wide ranging as meningococcal septicaemia, cystic fibrosis, congenital heart disease and diabetic ketoacidosis.

1.1 Anatomy

Lobes

The lungs are divided into lobes separated by fissures. The right lung has three anatomical lobes – the upper, middle and lower lobes. In contrast, the left lung has only two lobes – the upper and lower lobes. Although not divided by fissures, the left upper lobe is divided anatomically into an upper division corresponding anatomically to the right upper lobe and a lower or lingular division analogous to the right middle lobe.

Airways

The bronchial tree

The bronchial tree starts at the division of the trachea into right and left main bronchi (**Figure 1.1**). It divides up to 28 times from the trachea to the alveoli, the site of gaseous exchange between the air and the blood. It consists of the:

- Trachea
- Main bronchi, left and right
- Lobar bronchi, each supplying a lobe of the lung

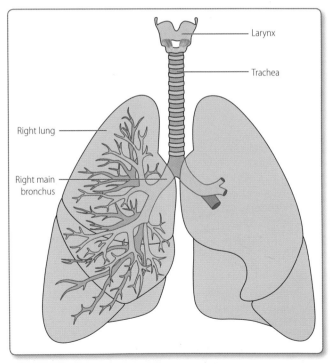

Figure 1.1 The bronchial tree (detail shown for the right lung only).

- Segmental bronchi, each supplying air to a bronchopulmonary segment (**Figure 1.2**)
- Lobular bronchi
- Conducting bronchioles
- Terminal bronchioles
- Respiratory bronchioles
- Alveolar ducts

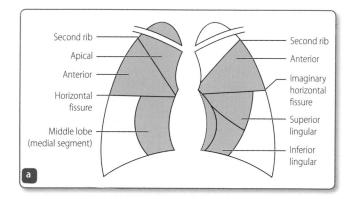

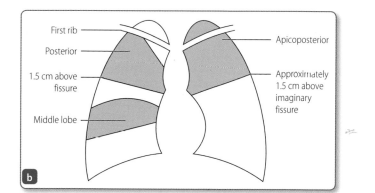

Figure 1.2 Posteroanterior views of the chest showing different pulmonary segments on each side. (a) Anterior view: note that there is no horizontal fissure on the left side, although an imaginary one has been drawn for convenience. The most median point on each side is the hilum. (b) Posterior view.

- Alveolar sacs
- Alveoli

No gaseous exchange takes place in the trachea and bronchi: they act as a pathway for air entering and leaving the lungs and have no other respiratory function.

Each bronchopulmonary segment is supplied by its own artery and is therefore a discrete anatomical and functional unit with respect to circulation as well as respiration. Bronchopulmonary segments are separated by connective tissue, with 10 segments in the right lung, and 8–10 in the left.

Each bronchopulmonary segment is anatomically divided into subsegments of various orders, down to the level of the lung **lobule (Figure 1.3)**. The lobule consists of a respiratory bronchiole and its first, second and third divisions, which continue as alveolar ducts, each duct terminating in an alveolar sac. The alveolar sac is a collection of alveoli separated partially or completely by connective tissue containing blood vessels, lymphatics and nerves.

Clinical insight

Pulmonary **surfactant** is a phospholipoprotein produced by type 2 alveolar cells. Like a detergent, it decreases surface tension within the alveoli, which increases the ability of the lungs to expand on inspiration and prevents lung collapse on exhalation.

Alveoli

The alveolar walls are lined by flat squamous cells on a basement membrane. This **respiratory membrane** is the site of gas exchange – diffusion between alveoli and capillary vessels. The structure of the respiratory membrane optimises gas exchange, and consists of:

- fluid/surfactant (keeping the alveoli patent)
- alveolar epithelial cells (95% are type I pneumocytes)
- epithelial basement membrane (structural network proteins)
- interstitial space (fluid)
- pulmonary capillary basement membrane
- capillary endothelium

The membrane itself is extremely thin (averaging 0.5 μm) with a large total surface area of about 55 m^2 provided by 700 million alveoli.

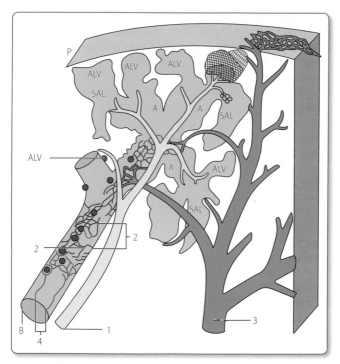

Figure 1.3 Primary respiratory lobule: subdivisions of the bronchial tree, pulmonary artery and vein. A, atria; ALV, alveoli along respiratory bronchiole and alveolar ducts; B, respiratory bronchiole which divides into two alveolar ducts; P, pleura; SAL, alveolar saccules; 1, pulmonary artery; 2, branches of pulmonary artery; 3, pulmonary vein; 4, bronchial arteries.

During normal inspiration, about two-thirds of the inhaled air enters the alveoli, the rest remaining in the 'anatomical dead space' of the conducting airways.

Pulmonary vasculature

Arteries

The lungs are supplied by two sets of arteries with distinct roles:

- **Pulmonary arteries,** which carry deoxygenated blood to receive oxygen from the alveoli (these are the only arteries in the body that carry deoxygenated blood)
- **Bronchial arteries,** which originate from the thoracic aorta and carry oxygenated blood to nourish the lung tissue

Pulmonary arteries accompany the bronchi, terminating in the pulmonary arterioles. These divide into dense capillary networks closely surrounding the alveolar walls. Bronchial arteries are relatively small and accompany the divisions of the bronchi.

Veins

The pulmonary veins arise chiefly from alveolar capillaries and, to a lesser extent, from other parts of the respiratory lobule and pleura. The ends of the veins coalesce into larger branches that follow a course independent of the bronchi and arteries. They are generally intersegmental, finally forming the four pulmonary veins (two from each lung) that empty oxygen-rich blood into the left atrium of the heart.

Most of the deoxygenated blood from lung tissue (non-alveolar capillary beds) returns to the heart via pulmonary veins; the rest joins the systemic deoxygenated blood in the azygos and hemiazygos veins via the bronchial veins.

1.2 Physiology

The primary purpose of the lungs is to provide an optimal and large surface area of respiratory membrane across which gaseous exchange occurs, with oxygen entering the blood and carbon dioxide being excreted from it. Successful gas exchange also requires that sufficient air is delivered to this membrane and, similarly, that blood flow to the capillary meshes surrounding the alveoli is adequate.

Clinical insight

Vital capacity varies greatly between people, usually between 3 and 5 L, and is therefore limited in its use in comparing lung function. However, a VC < 15 mL/kg is an indication for intubation and ventilatory support.

Lung volume

The important measurements of lung volume are shown in **Figure 1.4**.

While at rest, a healthy individual breathes in or out 400 mL air; this is the tidal volume (V_T). Over and above this tidal volume, an additional amount of about 2800 mL air can be breathed in by maximum effort; this is the **inspiratory reserve volume** (IRV). The sum total of tidal volume and inspiratory reserve volume, about 3200 mL, is the **inspiratory capacity** (IC).

The IRV is a measure of the reserve available to the individual for increase of tidal volume for exercise. Similarly after a normal expiration of tidal volume, it is possible to breathe out an amount of air equal to about 800 mL by maximal expiration called the **expiratory reserve volume** (ERV).

Vital capacity (VC) measures the maximum volume of air that can be breathed out after a maximal inspiration. In healthy individuals the VC is about 4000 mL. About 1000 mL of air remains inside the lungs even at the end of maximal expiration

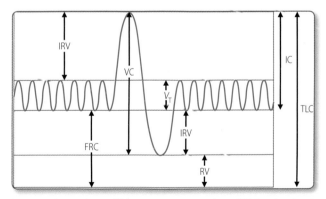

Figure 1.4 Lung volumes. ERV, expiratory reserve volume; FRC, functional residual capacity; IC, inspiratory capacity; IRV, inspiratory reserve volume; RV, residual volume; TLC, total lung capacity; V_T, tidal volume; VC, vital capacity.

because of negative intrathoracic pressure. This so-called **dead space** is termed the **residual volume** (RV).

The **total lung capacity** (TLC) is the total volume of gas contained in the lungs at the end of maximal inspiration:

TLC = VC + RV.

TLC is about 5 L in a healthy adult..

Breathing and lung compliance

Effective respiration requires that the lungs, pleurae and thoracic cavity are able to expand and contract to fully allow the inspiration and expiration of air. This ability to stretch in response to a change in pressure is termed lung compliance. It is dependent on the elastic forces of the lungs and thorax – in other words, how easy it is to increase their volume.

Guiding principle

Gas tensions in the blood are stated as **partial pressures**, measured in pascals (Pa) (previously mmHg – millimetres of mercury):

- In a mixture of ideal gases occupying a particular volume, the partial pressure of a single gas is the pressure that it would have if it occupied the volume alone (assuming stable pressure and temperature)
- Partial pressure is useful physiologically when discussing respiratory gases because it is the partial pressure that determines how gases diffuse between compartments, not the concentration
- Concentration is not the main 'driving force' for gas movement because gases can be immobilised by binding to molecules in body fluids (e.g. O_2 binds to haemoglobin), or they can be altered to another form (e.g. CO_2 reacts with water to form bicarbonate, HCO_3^-)

Respiration rate

A mechanical effort (the 'work of breathing') is required to move the lungs and related tissues. The rate and depth of respiration automatically adjust to produce the required alveolar ventilation, whether in a healthy or diseased state. As the rate increases, the depth decreases, and vice versa. Generally 10–14 respirations/min is the optimal rate in healthy adults.

Compliance

The work of breathing may be estimated indirectly by measuring the oxygen use during quiet breathing and during hyperventilation.

Direct determinations of the mechanical work of respiration may also be made, as discussed in Chapter 2. In practice, the clinical utility of measuring compliance is limited and measurements are undertaken only under certain circumstances to aid with long-term respiratory management, for example in an intensive care unit (ICU) for ventilated patients with pulmonary oedema or acute respiratory distress syndrome (ARDS) where abnormal compliance may result in difficulties in mechanical ventilation.

Neurological control of breathing

The primary function of the respiratory system is to maintain the oxygen (O_2) and carbon dioxide (CO_2) gas tensions of arterial blood (PaO_2 and $PaCO_2$) within narrow physiological limits suited to the body and its cells (**Table 1.1**). This is done through a number of mechanisms, all of which are controlled by the nervous system.

Clinical insight

In chronic hypoxic states such as chronic obstructive pulmonary disease (COPD) there is 'poisoning' of the central chemoreceptors of the medulla, because the main respiratory stimulus is continually the hypoxic drive via the peripheral chemoreceptors. Losing this sensitivity to CO_2 can have a dangerous effect if the hypoxia is corrected with oxygen therapy; they lose their stimulus and therefore under-ventilate, causing a build-up of CO_2 within about 20 min. A rise of $PaCO_2 > 6.5$ kPa may cause depressed mental function.

Gas	Atmospheric kPa (mmHg)	Alveolar kPa (mmHg)	Arterial kPa (mmHg)	Venous kPa (mmHg)
Oxygen	21.2 (159)	13.8 (104)	12.6 (95)	5.3 (40)
Carbon dioxide	0.03 (0.2)	5.3 (40)	5.3 (40)	6.1 (46)
Nitrogen	79.2 (596)	75.7 (569)	75.5 (568)	75.4 (567)
Water vapour	0.64 (4.8)	6.25 (47)	6.25 (47)	6.25 (47)
Total pressure	101.1 (760)	101.1 (760)	99.7 (750)	93.1 (700)

Table 1.1 Total and partial pressures of respiratory gases at sea level.

The act of breathing air in and out of the lungs is primarily controlled by the central nervous system. Receptors in the brain and the heart detect levels of O_2 and CO_2 and send signals to the lungs to adjust the level of respiration to compensate. These signals constitute the 'urge to breathe' and are known as the **respiratory drive**. CO_2 is the most important stimulus for respiration:

- Receptors for CO_2 are found in the medulla of the brain (central chemoreceptors)
- Receptors for O_2 are found mainly in carotid and aortic bodies (peripheral chemoreceptors; **Figure 1.5**).

CO_2 is the more important gas as the body has more capacity to store CO_2 than O_2 or hydrogen ions (H^+).

In normal people at sea level, only 10% of the respiratory drive is due to hypoxic stimulation. Unlike the central stimulation of hypercapnia, hypoxia causes central depression of the respiratory drive. Complete cessation of breathing for 1 minute causes a mild rise of $PaCO_2$ by 10 mmHg (1.3 kPa), whereas a dramatic drop in PaO_2 of 50 mmHg (6.5 kPa) occurs.

Respiratory drive is also influenced by blood pH. Hydrogen ions (H^+) stimulate both central receptors in the medulla

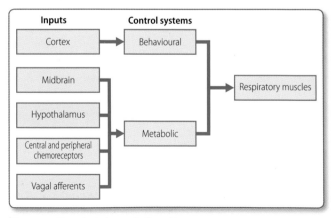

Figure 1.5 Neurological control of breathing.

and peripheral chemoreceptors in the carotid and aortic bodies, increasing respiratory drive. Acidosis (high H^+/low blood pH) stimulates respiration; conversely alkalosis depresses it. It is difficult to separate this influence from that of O_2 and CO_2.

Gas exchange: ventilation, diffusion and perfusion

The correct levels and balance of respiratory gases in the blood are vitally important to ensure adequate oxygen supply to the body and that CO_2 is excreted before it causes toxicity. Ordinarily the rate, depth and rhythm of breathing are precisely adjusted to the changing needs for O_2 uptake and CO_2 elimination so that the arterial blood tensions of these gases are maintained within normal limits despite wide variations in physical activity. The three main factors that are regulated to maintain this balance are: ventilation of the lungs (ventilation), gas crossing the respiratory membrane (diffusion) and gas exchange from the lungs to the blood circulation (perfusion) (**Figure 1.6**).

1. **Ventilation** is the drawing in of atmospheric air to reach the alveoli (inspiration) and removal of gases back to air (expiration). O_2 and CO_2 are then exchanged in the alveoli with O_2 diffusing into the bloodstream where it is available for cellular gas exchange. CO_2 produced by cells takes the reverse route, travelling in the bloodstream and later diffusing into the alveoli and then the outside air. In ventilation, the lungs act as a pair of bellows. Normal ventilation is dependent on four factors:

   (i)   an intact neuromuscular mechanism
   (ii) unrestricted movement of the chest wall and pleura
   (iii) distensible lungs
   (iv) patent airways

2. **Diffusion** is the process of gas exchange between alveoli and blood; for this the lungs provide an interface of total surface area about 55 m^2 via 700 million alveoli; O_2 passes across this alveolar–capillary membrane from the alveolar space to pulmonary capillary blood and CO_2 from capillaries to alveoli

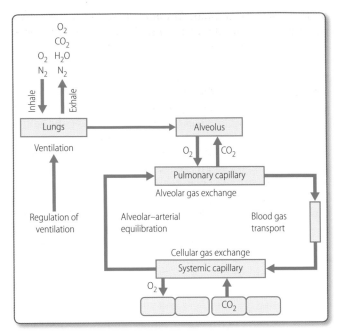

Figure 1.6 Processes involved in maintaining the correct levels of respiratory gases in the blood.

3. **Perfusion** of blood to the respiratory membrane must be enough to allow diffusion of gases and their transport into general circulation to meet the body's needs

The processes of ventilation, diffusion and perfusion are intimately linked in healthy individuals, but disease may affect any or all of them. It is critical to consider all three processes separately when trying to diagnose the exact cause of respiratory compromise in a patient.

Disorders affecting ventilation are the most common causes of compromised lung function in clinical practice. Disturbances of gas exchange are relatively far less frequent. Disorders of perfusion are common and can be fatal, e.g. a large pulmonary embolus. Testing ventilation is also much more straightforward than testing diffusion and is therefore more commonly done.

Alveolar ventilation

Alveolar ventilation is the volume of gas per unit time (L/min) that reaches the alveoli **(Figure 1.7)**. 'Alveolar ventilation' is that part of the total ventilation (i.e. all gas entering the lungs) that participates in gas exchange with pulmonary capillary blood; it is equal to total ventilation minus the ventilation of the conducting airways (i.e. dead-space ventilation).

The concept of alveolar ventilation is key to respiration because only gas reaching the alveoli can diffuse into the bloodstream. It is therefore important to determine how much inspired gas reaches the alveoli and how it is distributed between the alveoli. Any disorder of **alveolar ventilation** will mean that there is inappropriate gas exchange between the lung and blood, leading to major problems. Accordingly, two

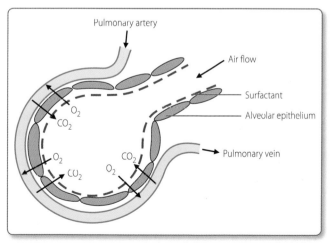

Figure 1.7 Alveolar ventilation.

factors need to be considered in alveolar ventilation: the volume and the distribution of gaseous exchange.

Volume of gaseous exchange

Alveolar ventilation ($\dot{V}_A$) is calculated by:
- the respiratory rate in breaths per minute
- the tidal volume (V_T) in millilitres – the amount of air that a healthy person breathes in or out in a normal breath
- the volume of the conducting airways in millilitres – the 'anatomical' dead space of the trachea and bronchi that does not take part in gas exchange. The dead space is fairly constant at approximately 180 mL in healthy males and 120 mL in healthy females

Alveolar ventilation in a healthy male is expressed (in L/min) as:

$$(\text{Tidal volume} - 180 \text{ mL}) \times \text{Respiratory rate.}$$

Accordingly, alveolar ventilation in a healthy female is expressed (in L/min) as:

$$(\text{Tidal volume} - 120 \text{ mL}) \times \text{Respiratory rate.}$$

The average alveolar ventilation is about 4 L/min.

Absolute values for alveolar ventilation are very difficult to measure in clinical practice. Rather, an indirect measure of alveolar ventilation is obtained by measurement of the PCO_2 (analogous to the measurement of oxygen tension as detailed above) of alveolar gas or arterial blood ($PaCO_2$). $PaCO_2$ is used as an index of alveolar ventilation because the alveolar and arterial PCO_2 values are almost identical and have a direct relationship, assuming that the respiratory membrane separating them is competent.

> ### Clinical insight
>
> Disturbances in distribution of alveolar air are marked in diseases where there is bronchial obstruction or emphysema (due to the mix of diseased and healthy lung tissue) or where there are uneven movements of the thoracic cage.

Distribution of alveolar air

Even if alveolar ventilation is normal, full arterial O_2 saturation may not be maintained if the inspired air is unevenly distributed among the functioning alveoli. The distribution of the inspired gas may vary in quantity within the alveoli at different times of the normal ventilatory cycle of inspiration followed by expiration, as even in the diseased state, when the anatomy of the lung is markedly uneven, pulmonary insufficiency may occur.

Alveolar ventilation and gas exchange

Alveolar ventilation is relatively constant in most people, because healthy lungs vary little anatomically or physically.

Alveolar ventilation influences gas exchange. The P_aCO_2 in arterial blood is directly related to the amount of CO_2 produced in the lungs per minute ($\dot{V}CO_2$) (i.e. a rise in $\dot{V}CO_2$ is associated with a rise in P_aCO_2). Conversely, P_aCO_2 is inversely proportional to alveolar ventilation, and so consequently:

- When alveolar ventilation increases, the P_aCO_2 falls
- When alveolar ventilation decreases, P_aCO_2 rises, which explains the rise in P_aCO_2 when patients have reduced or impaired ventilation.

Alveolar oxygen tension

The alveolar oxygen tension the partial pressure of oxygen within the alveoli (P_AO_2). It is one factor that influences the diffusion of gases across the alveolar–capillary membrane. It can be determined through the laboratory analysis of an end-tidal sample of expired air (see Chapter 2) or calculated at sea level (without the need for collection of expired air, which can be quite cumbersome) from the following equation:

$$P_AO_2 = F_iO_2 \times (P_B - PH_2O) - P_aCO_2/R$$

where F_iO_2 is the fraction of inspired air (21%), P_B the barometric pressure (760 mmHg), PH_2O is the pressure of water vapour in air (47 mmHg at 37°C when fully saturated) and R is the respiratory quotient (normal range is 0.6–0.9), which is a unitless number used for a range of calculations of basal metabolic rate.

Alveolar–capillary diffusion

Alveolar–capillary diffusion is the process of gas exchange within the alveoli; it is crucial to determining how much O_2 reaches the blood.

O_2 moves from the alveolar space, through the respiratory membrane and blood plasma, and into the erythrocyte by diffusion down its pressure gradient, i.e. from higher to lower PO_2. Any disturbance in the respiratory membrane may impair oxygen diffusion. CO_2 diffuses from blood to alveolar air. As CO_2 has a diffusing capacity that is about 20 times greater than that of O_2, impairment of its diffusion is of theoretical interest only.

The **diffusing capacity** of O_2 is a measurement of the ability of the respiratory membrane to transfer O_2. It is calculated as the volume of O_2 (mL) that diffuses across the alveolar–capillary membrane per minute per mmHg mean pressure difference (i.e. the pressure gradient). In practice, alveolar–capillary diffusion is measured by calculating the resting diffusing capacity of carbon monoxide (see Chapter 2 for more details on how this is measured).

Gas exchange in the lungs

Gas exchange is the process by which oxygen moves from the alveoli into the bloodstream and carbon dioxide moves in the opposite direction. The three key clinical determinants of gas exchange are:
1. Ventilation–perfusion quotient ($\dot{V}/\dot{Q}$)
2. Alveolar–arterial oxygen gradient ($P_{A-a}O_2$)
3. Shunt component ($\dot{Q}_S/\dot{Q}_T$)

Ventilation–perfusion ratio

The ventilation–perfusion ratio (or quotient) is a measure of how much of the O_2 that enters the alveoli is moved into the blood. This parameter is important because a number of diseases can alter this value, leading to problems with low blood oxygen and hence tissue hypoxia despite adequate O_2 making it to the lungs (see Chapter 3 for more details).

The basic function of the lungs is to transfer the quantity of O_2, from inspired air to arterial blood, that the body tissues need and to remove from the venous blood the amount of CO_2 produced by metabolism. The total quantities of gases transferred depend on the amount of air that arrives in the alveoli ($\dot{V}_A$ – ventilation of the alveoli) and overall perfusion of the pulmonary capillaries ($\dot{Q}_c$), which in turn depends on the cardiac output.

The normal ventilation–perfusion ratio ($\dot{V}/\dot{Q}$ ratio) is calculated as follows:

$$\frac{\dot{V}_A}{\dot{Q}_c} = \frac{\text{Pulmonary alveolar ventilation (L/min)}}{\text{Pulmonary capillary perfusion (L/min)}}$$

The average alveolar ventilation is about 4 L/min, and the average normal blood flow through the lungs is about 5 L/min, giving a ventilation–perfusion quotient of 0.8.

Alveolar–arterial oxygen gradient

The alveolar–arterial oxygen gradient ($P_{A-a}O_2$) is a measure of the oxygen that has reached the arterial blood supply as a ratio of the total oxygen in the alveoli. It is a useful index of pulmonary gas exchange function. This requires that three elements are working correctly:

- *Circulatory anatomy is normal.* Anomalies such as congenital heart defects (atrial septal defect, patent ductus arteriosus) cause **anatomical shunting,** i.e. venous blood passes through routes that are not exposed to alveolar air
- *Ventilation and perfusion are matched* so that ventilated areas of the lung are matched by venous blood perfusion. A mismatch is termed **functional shunting** in that there is an imbalance between the supply of air and the supply of blood to certain regions of the lungs. For example, collapse of a lung does not provide ventilation to perfused blood in the collapsed region and is tantamount to a shunt, and pulmonary arterial occlusion will not provide perfusion to a normally ventilated region
- *The respiratory membrane allows sufficient free diffusion of gases between air and blood.* A diffusion defect impairs the alveolar–capillary membrane, e.g. in interstitial lung fibrosis

Real-time measurement of the $P_{A-a}O_2$ requires simultaneous measurement of P_AO_2 and P_aO_2. To measure the $P_{A-a}O_2$ the alveolar oxygen tension is measured or calculated as previously described and an arterial blood sample is simultaneously collected for ABG analysis, giving the P_AO_2, P_aO_2, P_ACO_2 and P_aCO_2. The $P_{A-a}O_2$ is important clinically in disease diagnosis, to assess disease severity and response to mechanical ventilators and O_2 therapy.

Shunt component

The shunt component is a measure of the proportion of venous blood that bypasses the respiratory membrane. In normal lungs there is a small amount of shunting of pulmonary arterial blood to the pulmonary veins; this is caused by:

- Direct arteriovenous communication
- Veins draining into the left ventricle
- Alveoli that have no ventilation, resulting in a direct shunt

In a healthy individual breathing room air (at F_iO_2 21) the PO_2 in alveolar air is 104 mmHg (13.8 kPa) and in arterial blood 95 mmHg (12.6 kPa). P_AO_2 exceeds P_aO_2 by 15 mmHg (2 kPa). Thus, at an F_iO_2 of 21, the $P_{A-a}O_2$ is 15 mmHg (2 kPa).

On breathing 100% O_2 ($F_iO_2 = 100$) enough O_2 will be supplied to saturate all the blood, leaving alveolar–capillary exchange areas, so the simplified equation for absolute shunt ($\dot{Q}_S/\dot{Q}_T$) is

$$\frac{\dot{Q}_S}{\dot{Q}_T} = \frac{(P_AO_2 - P_aO_2) \times (0.003)}{4 + (P_AO_2 - P_aO_2) \times (0.003)}$$

where the constant 4 is the assumed arteriovenous difference in volume %, and 0.003 is the solubility coefficient of oxygen in plasma at 37°C.

The shunt fraction is clinically useful in critical care monitoring as abnormalities in the fraction in patients who are intubated and ventilated may reveal underlying problems such as ventilation – perfusion imbalances or atelectasis in the lungs. The normal shunt fraction is less than 5%.

Clinical insight

Causes of increased pulmonary blood pressure include:

- COPD
- interstitial lung disease
- thoracic cage deformities
- sleep apnoea
- intravascular thromboembolism
- vasculitis

Pulmonary blood flow

The output of the right ventricle is about 5–6 L/min in a resting healthy adult and flows directly into the pulmonary circulation. The pulmonary arterial pressure is about 15–30 mmHg during systole and 5–10 mmHg during diastole. The channels of flow are large, and the resistance is about a fifth of that of the systemic circulation. The blood flow during exercise may increase sixfold to about 30 L/min, with a slight increase in pressure.

Perfusion

Pulmonary arterial pressure is low at the apex and high at the base of the lungs because the blood flow is greater when it has less work to do against gravity. Consequently, oxygen perfusion (i.e. the amount of oxygen reaching the blood from the lungs) is also lowest at the lung apex and highest at the lung base. During exercise, the increase in cardiac output causes the pulmonary vasculature to vasodilate, leading to increased pulmonary perfusion without a raise in mean arterial pressure.

Pulmonary vascular resistance

This is the pressure against which blood in the pulmonary circulation has to flow and can be obtained from pulmonary arterial pressure, pulmonary capillary wedge pressure (an estimate of pulmonary capillary bed pressure) and cardiac output. The resistance increases when pulmonary arterial and arteriolar vasoconstriction occurs in alveolar hypoxia and this is seen in a number of different lung diseases. More prolonged and severe alveolar hypoxia leads to increased resistance and raised pulmonary blood pressure.

O_2 and CO_2 transport by the blood

The transport of gases in the blood is crucial to maintaining a normal metabolic state. O_2 is used up by cells in respiration and the product, CO_2, needs to then be transported back to the lungs to be breathed out in exchange for more O_2. Abnormalities in this process will lead to changes in metabolism and acid–base status which can be measured by arterial blood gas analysis (see Chapters 2 and 3).

Guiding principle

There are three main measurements of arterial oxygen:

- **Oxygen content (P_aO_2)** is the pressure of oxygen molecules dissolved in blood, and is measured by ABG analysis with units of kPa or mmHg
- **Oxygen saturation (S_aO_2)** is a measure of the percentage of haemoglobin sites that have oxygen bound, commonly measured with a pulse oximeter
- **Oxygen content (C_aO_2)** is the real measure of blood oxygen quantity as it accounts for dissolved and haemoglobin-bound oxygen. It is given as the volume of oxygen carried in each 100 ml blood (mL O_2/100 mL), and is normally 15-20 ml/100 ml

Oxygen

Oxygen saturation (S_aO_2) is to the percentage of haemoglobin-binding sites that are occupied by oxygen, thereby forming oxyhaemoglobin. Arterial blood is normally at 97–98% O_2 saturation (i.e. 98% of the available haemoglobin is combined with O_2), whereas venous blood is normally at 74% O_2 saturation.

As blood flows through tissues in which the PO_2 is lower than in arterial blood, O_2 diffuses into the tissues. Under resting conditions, the O_2 saturation falls to about 74% in venous blood being returned to the lungs. When venous blood is exposed to the higher PO_2 in the alveoli, there is a diffusion of O_2 into the blood across the alveolar membrane.

O_2 constitutes 21% of the atmosphere by volume and atmospheric PO_2 is 159 mmHg at sea level (**Figure 1.8**). At an alveolar pressure of 104 mmHg, alveolar oxygen diffuses into pulmonary

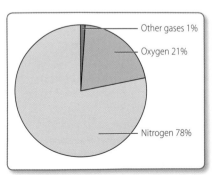

Other gases 1%

Oxygen 21%

Nitrogen 78%

Figure 1.8 Composition of atmospheric gases.

venous blood and raises its O_2 content from 15 mL/100 mL to 20 mL/100 mL. Of this amount 19.75 mL is combined with haemoglobin and 0.25 mL is 'free' or dissolved in simple solution in the plasma. At this pressure of alveolar O_2, haemoglobin in the arterial blood normally becomes 98% saturated and 2% of the haemoglobin remains reduced, i.e. free of oxygen.

The O_2-binding capacity of haemoglobin is influenced by the CO_2 content and pH of blood (**Figure 1.9**). Increased PCO_2 causes dissociation of O_2 from oxyhaemoglobin because haemoglobin has a higher affinity for CO_2 than O_2. From the alveolar capillaries, CO_2 diffuses freely into alveolar air, lowering the CO_2 content of the blood and permitting haemoglobin to bind more O_2.

Carbon dioxide

In blood, CO_2 is present in both plasma and erythrocytes:
- Dissolved in blood plasma (5.3% in arterial blood)
- Bound to haemoglobin as carbaminohaemoglobin within erythrocytes (4.5%)
- In the form of bicarbonate attached to a base (90%)

As CO_2 diffuses from peripheral tissues into blood plasma, some of it hydrates slowly to carbonic acid. Most of the CO_2,

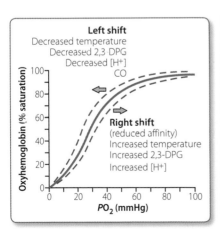

Left shift
Decreased temperature
Decreased 2,3-DPG
Decreased [H+]
CO

Right shift
(reduced affinity)
Increased temperature
Increased 2,3-DPG
Increased [H+]

Oxyhemoglobin (% saturation) — vertical axis: 0, 20, 40, 60, 80, 100

PO_2 (mmHg) — horizontal axis: 0, 20, 40, 60, 80, 100

Figure 1.9 Haemoglobin saturation curve. In the normal state, the solid line reflects the affinity of haemoglobin for oxygen. Factors that decrease this affinity cause a 'right shift' in the curve, whereas those that increase this affinity (i.e. oxygen is bound more readily) cause a 'left shift' in the curve. 2,3-DPG, 2,3-diphosphoglycerate, a byproduct of cell metabolism that stabilises deoxyhaemoglobin.

however, passes preferentially into erythrocytes, where some of it combines with haemoglobin to form carbaminohaemoglobin.

Most of the CO_2 entering red blood cells is rapidly hydrated by the enzyme carbonic anhydrase to carbonic acid, which immediately dissociates to form bicarbonate (**Figure 1.10**). This enzyme is therefore essential in regulating blood and body fluid pH and transporting CO_2 out of tissues. The process of bicarbonate formation increases as haemoglobin loses oxygen. The bicarbonate ions then diffuse into the plasma and chloride ions diffuse into the erythrocytes until equilibrium is established.

pH homeostasis

Cells are continually producing acid as a consequence of metabolism. Because most proteins and enzymes require an environment with a pH of 7.35–7.45 in order to function effectively, it is important that pH is tightly controlled and that this tendency to acidosis is countered. The normal pH of blood (7.40) is maintained by the gain or loss of H^+ or HCO_3^- by three mechanisms:

- **Plasma buffer system** – the most important element in this is the carbonic acid–bicarbonate system (**Figure 1.10**), shown as the equation $H_2O + CO_2 \leftrightarrow H_2CO_3 \leftrightarrow HCO_3^- + H^+$
- **Alveolar ventilation** – the excretion of waste CO_2 in the lungs
- **Renal regulation** – the excretion of protons (H^+) by the kidneys

Key to understanding pH homeostasis is to remember that these three mechanisms of acid–base balance (carbonic acid

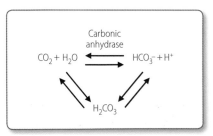

Figure 1.10 Carbonic anhydrase, the key buffering system of plasma pH homeostasis.

buffering, CO_2 excretion and renal H^+ excretion) are closely intertwined in healthy individuals.

The carbonic acid–bicarbonate equation is central to this homeostasis, but the direction of the equation in which the reaction is driven is dependent on excretion of CO_2 and H^+ from the blood. This means that the plasma can buffer initial acid or base changes that occur, but it has its limits. The system (i.e. the blood) is not closed: the excess CO_2 and H^+ can be excreted by the lungs and the kidneys, respectively. This is known as **compensation**.

> ### Guiding principle
>
> A buffer, such as carbonic acid, is a chemical that can compensate for changes in pH. The carbonic acid–bicarbonate system is catalysed by carbonic anhydrase.

Acid generated by metabolism is either excreted in the lungs (as exhaled CO_2) or kidneys (as H^+ in urine) or is neutralised by regeneration of bicarbonate (HCO_3^-). The kidneys excrete less than 1% of the carbon dioxide in the form of carbonic acid and the remaining carbon dioxide is removed via the lungs.

The pH is determined by the ratio of plasma bicarbonate to dissolved carbon dioxide in blood [($HCO_3^-/[H_2CO_3]$)] which is about 20:1. This homeostatic ratio is normally maintained by alveolar ventilation. When the CO_2 pressure rises in the blood, the respiratory centre is stimulated, increasing alveolar ventilation and blowing off excess CO_2, returning its partial pressure to normal.

Base excess

The base excess is the theoretical amount of acid needed to bring a patient's fully oxygenated blood to normal blood pH at room temperature (pH 7.40). It is calculated from the serum bicarbonate concentration [(HCO_3^-)] and pH: the normal base excess is between –2 and +2 mmol/L. It can be used as a rapid indication of a patient's metabolic state. A high base excess (i.e. above +2 mmol/L) is metabolic alkalosis, whereas a low one (below –2 mmol/L) represents metabolic acidosis. The **standard base excess** is the base excess when haemoglobin is at 5 g/dL, and is clinically a more useful estimate of extracellular fluid pH.

Anion gap

The anion gap is the difference between the total sodium and potassium ion plasma concentrations and the total chloride and bicarbonate plasma concentrations (in mmol/L):

$$\text{Anion gap} = ([Na^+] + [K^+]) - ([HCO_3^-] + [Cl^-])$$

It provides an indication of how much unmeasured ions are contributing to acidosis, and therefore can help elucidate its cause.

The normal range is 10–18 mmol/L (see Chapter 3). Assessment of the anion gap is useful in cases of metabolic acidosis, to help in diagnosing the underlying cause. Although the differential diagnosis is wide, in general:

- **A high anion gap** indicates ingestion or production of too much acid, most often from lactic acidosis
- **A low/normal anion gap** indicates that excessive bicarbonate is being lost by the gastrointestinal tract (e.g. diarrhoea) or due to tubular damage in distal (type 1) or proximal (type 2) renal tubular acidosis

Physiological changes during exercise

Cardiac changes during exercise

Physical activity is associated with changes in:
- cardiac output
- stroke volume
- heart rate
- systemic and pulmonary blood pressure
- the microcirculation
- regional blood flow

Cardiac output and stroke volume

During the first phase of a rhythmic muscle exercise, there is a sudden initial rise in the cardiac output, followed by a slow increase to a level required by the intensity of the exercise. This level is reached when the O_2 consumption is at a steady state.

Healthy individuals can adjust their cardiac output faster than those who are unhealthy. During muscular activity for a relatively short effort, the stroke volume rises quickly to a level that remains constant. For a more prolonged effort the stroke volume can decrease by as much as 16%, but the heart rate increases to ensure that the cardiac output remains constant.

> ## Clinical insight
>
> The heart rate increases proportional to the severity of the workload but it increases more rapidly in an unhealthy person.

Heart rate
During heavy work the heart rate increases until a state of muscular exhaustion has been reached. The heart rate achieved at the steady state strictly relates directly to the O_2 uptake.

Blood pressure
During exercise the systolic blood pressure increases slightly for the initial 1–2 minutes despite the simultaneous dilatation of resistance vessels. The blood pressure subsequently stabilises for each workload at a particular level for each individual. The peripheral resistance falls during muscular activity due to extreme dilatation of the arterioles in muscles, and the pressure in the pulmonary arteries rises along with the cardiac output.

Perfusion
Only a portion of the capillary vascular bed is open at rest. During muscular activity the number of patent capillary vessels and the amount of blood flow increase by up to 20 times. Although the velocity of capillary flow does not change, the diffusion distance that molecules must travel from the blood to the cellular site of metabolic activity is considerably shortened.

Respiratory changes during exercise
The response of the respiratory system during physical activity is to provide adequate O_2 through ventilation and diffusion.

At rest, the lungs ventilate at a rate of 5–6 L/min. Ventilation increases during muscle work, according to metabolic demands, and during heavy activity can reach values of 20–25 times the level at rest. During muscular work the TLC decreases slightly, the VC is reduced and the RV rises a little. Although ventilation may increase dramatically during exercise, it imposes a relatively low energy cost.

Understanding the tests

Understanding normal patterns in both lung function and arterial blood gases (ABGs) facilitates a greater understanding of why things go wrong and how disease affects these investigations. ABG results allow rapid assessment of both the metabolic and the respiratory state. Knowledge of the physiological mechanisms behind pH measurement, electrolyte levels and haemoglobin oxygenation are key to interpreting a normal ABG.

A full understanding of the mechanics behind normal lung function is also key to interpreting abnormalities encountered in disease. The wide ranges of normal in both lung function and ABG testing should be taken into consideration when analysing both investigations.

2.1 Arterial blood gases

ABG analysis is an important test with substantial clinical utility for the diagnosis, management and monitoring of a number of respiratory and cardiac diseases. ABG results are usually presented as 'on room air', an approach followed in this book unless otherwise indicated. Blood gas analysis gives valuable information on a person's acid–base status, oxygenation and ventilation, and other physiological values. The main disadvantages of ABG analysis are that it is invasive and the results only give a 'snapshot' of the patient's status at one point in time. Physiological status can change rapidly, which is why continuous monitoring is needed in critically ill patients, e.g. through use of arterial lines.

Table 2.1 shows clinical situations that indicate when an ABG should be performed.

Clinical uses of ABG analysis are given in **Table 2.2** and the readings in normal young adults are given in **Table 2.3.** The

Scenario	Indication
Presentation	CO_2 retention: drowsy, CO_2 flapping tremor, headache, palmar redness, bounding pulse Hypoxia: cyanosis, confusion, hallucinations
Monitoring a critically ill patient	Respiratory failure A ventilated patient Serious trauma Post-surgery
Clinical decline	Acute exacerbation of chronic lung disease Impaired consciousness or respiratory effort Unexpected decline in a sick patient
Pulse oximetry verification	When values need to be checked

Table 2.1 When to perform an arterial blood gas (ABG).

Measurement	Example of clinical use
O_2 capacity of the lungs	A normal O_2 capacity would point away from a pulmonary embolus in a patient with risk factors and signs of a suspected blood clot in the lungs
O_2 pressure within the blood	A low level of blood oxygenation may be used as an indication of need for positive airway pressure in a patient with COPD who was not responding to O_2 via a facemask
Level of ventilation compared with body's needs	Low levels of O_2 or high levels of CO_2 in the blood may result in an increased level of ventilation for a patient undergoing a major operation
Acid–base status in the blood	The level of acidity in the blood of a patient with diabetic ketoacidosis will correlate with the severity of disease and need for critical care assessment
Electrolyte levels in the blood	Rapid assessment of potassium levels in a patient with acute renal failure

COPD, chronic obstructive pulmonary disease.

Table 2.2 Clinical uses of arterial blood gas parameters.

ABG measure	Level
pH	7.35–7.45
PO_2 (kPa)	10–13
PCO_2 (kPa)	4.5–6.0
Bicarbonate (mmol/L)	21–26
Base excess (mmol/L)	−2 to +2

Table 2.3 Normal arterial blood gas (ABG) results in a young adult.

principles behind the abnormalities seen in P_aO_2, P_aCO_2 and pH readings on and ABG are discussed in Chapter 3.

Taking ABG samples

For routine analysis, direct radial artery puncture with a 20-gauge needle, using a heparinised syringe to prevent immediate clotting, is generally the preferred technique (**Figures 2.1** and **2.2**). Other arteries of choice include the brachial and femoral vessels.

Procedure

Meticulous collection of the blood sample is essential.

1. Get all needed equipment ready: sharps bin, pre-heparinised syringe, 23-G (blue) needle, gloves, alcohol wipe, gauze, tape
2. Look and feel for the best site on both sides (radial artery at wrist is most common) and wipe site with alcohol, leaving to dry
3. The skin above the artery at the puncture site can be pre-anaesthetised with 1% lidocaine via a 25-G needle

Clinical insight

For ABG sampling:
- Get an expert to teach you arterial puncture
- Don't use the radial artery if there is an arteriovenous fistula for dialysis
- Explain to the patient that it will feel different to venepuncture

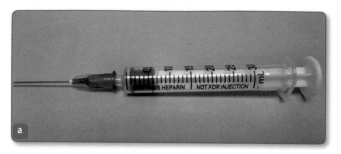

Figure 2.1 Taking arterial blood gases: (a) syringe and (b) machine.

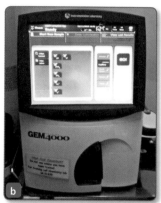

Figure 2.2 How to take an arterial blood gas.

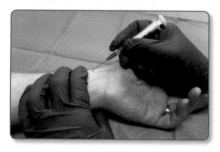

4. Hold the ABG syringe like a pen, getting a third person to hold the patient's arm with the wrist slightly extended. Feeling for the pulse with your free hand, enter needle at 45° with the bevel facing upwards, below your finger sensing the pulse

5. Let the syringe fill under the force of arterial pressure (this avoids air bubbles) until 1–2 mL is collected

6. Withdraw smoothly and quickly, immediately applying firm pressure to the puncture site with your free hand to prevent bruising

Guiding principle

- In the UK, ABGs are reported in kilopascals (kPa). In other regions, such as North America and the Indian subcontinent, millimetres of mercury (mmHg) are used instead.
- 1 kPa is equivalent to 7.5 mmHg
- 1 mmHg is equivalent to 0.133 kPa.

7. Air bubbles in the syringe should be immediately expelled if present

8. Mix the sample thoroughly by rolling the syringe between your palms

9. Ideally, analysis is immediate or within 2 hours, storing in a bag of ice

Electrolytes

A standard blood gas machine reports certain blood electrolyte levels as well as giving blood gas content. These usually include sodium and potassium, which can be helpful in emergency situations, e.g. a high potassium reading may help elucidate the cause of a cardiac arrest. More sophisticated machines also analyse, for example, methaemoglobin and carboxyhaemoglobin content.

2.2 Monitoring ABGs in ventilated and anaesthetised patients

Patients who are ventilated and in intensive care (either fully ventilated and sedated or conscious with a lower level of support such as continuous positive airway pressure) or who are anaesthetised and undergoing long and complex operations need regular arterial blood monitoring. This ensures that the level of ventilation that they receive is appropriate for their condition. Regular monitoring allows fine adjustments to be made to achieve ventilation.

Repeated ABG cannulation can cause local bruising and swelling, and can be extremely painful once the patient regains consciousness. More serious adverse events include the appearance of haematomas, nerve injury or limb ischaemia due to arterial occlusion.

For these reasons, patients who are to undergo repeated ABG measurements will often have a line placed within the artery from which blood can be drawn (**Figures 2.3** and **2.4**). In addition to the sampling of gases, an arterial line provides an accurate real-time measure of blood pressure, which is vital for a patient who is ventilated.

2.3   Lung function tests

Lung function tests (LFTs) are an important objective method of diagnosing respiratory impairment, quantifying its severity and evaluating the effectiveness of treatment. A number of different forms of lung function testing can be performed but the most common hospital test is spirometry, which provides **flow–volume loops:** graphs displaying different parameters of lung function.

The tests enable early detection of pulmonary insufficiency in many patients who may otherwise appear clinically and

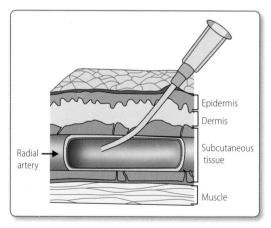

Figure 2.3 Placement of an arterial line.

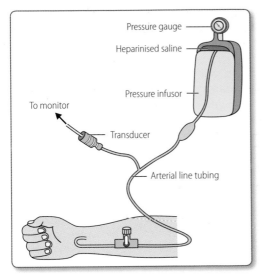

Figure 2.4 Arterial line set-up.

radiologically normal. They also provide a quantitative measurement of respiratory impairment, which is usually not obtainable by radiology or other methods. The tests can, for example, differentiate the breathlessness of cardiac origin from that of pulmonary origin, and can also differentiate between organic disease of the lung and functional symptoms that mimic a cardiorespiratory disorder. LFTs are also used to assess fitness for high altitude, air travel and diving. However, tests of respiratory function are not sufficiently specific to diagnose an individual disease with certainty. They are valuable in that they enable the practitioner to identify the contributions of ventilatory failure and diffusion defects, as well as to estimate the degree of respiratory failure present.

In industrial medicine, lung function tests are used to assess the degree of disability and the expectation of life due to occupational lung disease. They are also fundamental in the assessment of the immediate risks and ultimate expectation of

Clinical insight

Lung function testing is contraindicated in:

- pneumothorax
- suspected infectious respiratory disease, e.g. tuberculosis
- recent myocardial infarction or unstable angina
- vascular aneurysms
- recent surgery, e.g. ophthalmic surgery

life before and after thoracic surgery. However, the tests of respiratory function are not sufficiently specific to identify with certainty any individual disease. They are valuable in that they enable the practitioner to identify the contributions of ventilatory failure and diffusion defects as well as to estimate the degree of respiratory failure present.

Table 2.4 summarises the main parameters of lung function that are measured.

Peak expiratory flow

Peak expiratory flow (PEF) is the maximal flow (speed) that can be achieved during a maximally forced expiration (initiated

Acronym	Parameter	Definition
PEFR	Peak expiratory flow rate	Maximum speed of forced expiration
VC	Vital capacity	Maximum volume of air breathed out after maximum inspiration
FVC	Forced vital capacity	The total volume of a forced exhalation after a maximal inspiration
FEV_1	Forced expiratory volume in 1 second	Maximum volume of air breathed out in first second of an FVC manoeuvre
FET	Forced expiratory time	Time taken to forcibly exhale vital capacity
FEF	Forced expiratory flow	Speed of exhalation during FVC
FEF_{25-75}	Forced expiratory flow 25–75%	FEF between 25 and 75% of FVC
MVV	Maximal voluntary ventilation	Maximum volume of air breathed per minute

Table 2.4 Parameters measured by spirometry.

at full inspiration) and is measured in litres per minute. As well as being used to diagnose disease, it can be used to assess how well or unwell a patient is from a respiratory point of view.

PEF is measured with a peak flow meter (**Figure 2.5**), a small hand-held device measuring the speed at which a patient can exhale. It measures the rate of flow of air through the bronchi and therefore the amount of obstruction present. The reading is recorded as the peak expiratory flow rate (PEFR).

The correct technique for measuring PEFR is as follows:
- Try to use the same peak flow meter for the same patient to avoid variability between devices
- Ask the patient to stand up straight and hold the peak flow meter horizontally (**Figure 2.5**)
- The patient should take a deep breath in, place the lips around the device to form a tight seal and then blow as hard and as fast as possible

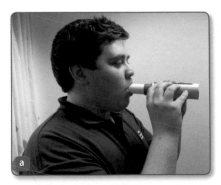
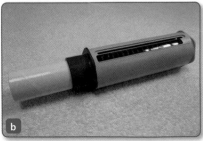

Figure 2.5 (a) The correct technique for measuring peak flow. (b) A typical peak flow meter, issued in the UK.

- The best of three consecutive readings should be taken as the result
- When used regularly the results can be recorded on a peak flow chart

There is a wide range of normal readings, and the expected PEFR is relative to a person's sex and height (**Figure 2.6**).

Peak flow charts

A number of different charts are used to record peak flow:

- The Wright scale
- The EN 13826 or EU scale (currently used in the UK) (**Figure 2.6**)
- The ATS (American Thoracic Society) scale

Peak flow readings may also be classified into three colour-coordinated zones (green, yellow and red), depending on

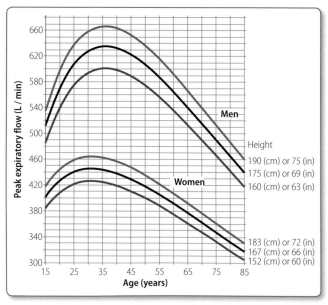

Figure 2.6 A typical peak flow chart used in the EU, showing a range of normal values based on gender, age and height.

the severity of disease. This allows for a standardised management protocol.

Spirometry

Spirometry is the most common method for testing overall pulmonary function. It enables rapid measurement of the amount and speed of air that is moved in and out of the lungs during breathing. Most hospitals and many primary health-care centres routinely perform spirometry, as it is an important investigation for assessing a number of cardiorespiratory diseases.

Spirometers range from hand-held electronic devices (**Figure 2.7**) to larger mechanical instruments. The results are presented as graphs (spirograms) which display information in two ways:

- **Volume–time curves** showing time on the x-axis and volume on the y-axis
- **Flow–volume loops** which show the rate of airflow on the y-axis and the total volume moving in or out of the lungs on the x-axis

Clinical insight

A single PEFR reading cannot be used alone to diagnose obstructive airway disease such as asthma, but regular multiple recordings showing a diurnal pattern may help diagnose the disease. Once diagnosed, PEFR readings are used to monitor disease severity and response to bronchodilators and steroids.

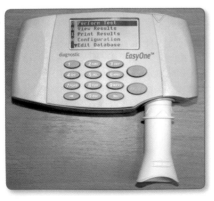

Figure 2.7 Electronic hand-held spirometer.

The results may be plotted on a graph or given as raw data, which are then interpreted against predicted results.

The usual procedure of measurement is as follows:

1. The patient is asked to take a deep breath and then exhale as strongly and for as long as possible into the mouthpiece

2. This may be followed by an immediate inhalation to investigate obstructive airway disease

3. Additional tests may involve soft breathing in and out (to calculate the tidal volume) or rapid inspiratory breaths (to calculate the forced expiration)

4. A bronchodilator may be given and the test may be repeated to measure the effect on lung function

5. Functional residual capacity may be measured using a plethysmograph or helium dilution test

> ## Clinical insight
>
> Check that the patient understands what the test involves, particularly that a good seal around the mouthpiece is needed and that breathing must be maximum effort:
>
> - Using the mouthpiece alone, get the patient to blow through it as a dummy run
>
> - Often patients expect some form of resistance and stop midway due to surprise; encourage them to blow as hard and for as long as they can (e.g. for 6 seconds or more)
>
> - If the patient coughs due to bulbar disease or has difficulty exhaling with force, try measuring *slow vital capacity* (SVC) first

Limitations of spirometry

Spirometry may not be suitable for patients with certain serious lung diseases and those who cannot understand the instructions, such as young children. Results may be unhelpful in patients with intermittent lung disease (e.g. mild asthma), when measurements may be deceptively normal. As the procedure is very patient dependent, reliable results require good patient technique.

Measurements of lung volume

For definitions of tidal volume (V_T), residual volume (RV) and vital capacity (VC), see Chapter 1.

Total lung capacity

The total volume of gas contained in the lungs at the end of maximal inspiration is equal to the VC plus RV, called the *total lung capacity* (TLC):

$$TLC = VC + RV.$$

It is about 5 L (see **Figure 1.4**). It can be measured by re-breathing helium through a closed circuit or by plethysmography using an airtight body box to measure total airflow.

These static measurements of TLC have limited clinical application compared with more dynamic ventilation tests. They are, however, useful when repeated at intervals to show an improvement or decline in lung function over time.

RV/TLC ratio

An important ratio is the residual volume to the total lung capacity ([RV/TLC] × 100). Normal values range from 20% to 35% in young people. This ratio tells you how much air is staying in the lungs after maximum exhalation, i.e. it is an indication of the level of 'gas trapping'. An increase may reflect a larger RV as in emphysema or a smaller TLC as in fibrosis. In older people, the ratio may be as high as 50%, with no apparent disability.

Residual volume can be calculated by deducting the expiratory reserve volume (ERV) from the functional residual capacity (FRC). FRC is the amount of air remaining in the lungs (especially in the parenchyma) after a passive expiration. So:

$$RV = FRC - ERV.$$

ERV is measured in normal spirometry, whereas FRC is usually measured in a closed-circuit helium dilution circuit. This involves using a spirometer containing a known volume and concentration of helium. The helium volume introduced and the final concentration of helium are read directly from kymographic records and a helium analyser meter. The FRC is calculated from the known initial and final volumes and the concentration of the gas. An alternative approach is to use a body plethysmographic method for measuring the resting end-expiratory thoracic gas volume (**Figure 2.8**).

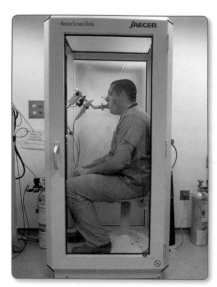

Figure 2.8 Body plethysmography.

Dynamic lung volume measurements

Dynamic tests of ventilation measure volumes breathed over a period of time. These are used to investigate dyspnoea, to differentiate between obstructive or restrictive disease, and to evaluate response to therapy. Common tests include resting minute ventilation, walking ventilation and maximum voluntary ventilation.

Resting minute ventilation

This is the total volume of air breathed in or out in 1 min while an individual is resting. It is about 5 L/min in a healthy individual. It can be calculated either by multiplying the tidal volume (V_T) by the respiratory rate (RR) or determined directly by spirometry. Resting minute ventilation (RMV) depends on V_T and RR. During exercise, ventilation is increased by increases in both rate and V_T. A better understanding of the performance of an individual can be obtained by comparing resting ventilation with the ventilation required for a given exercise.

Walking ventilation

Walking ventilation (WV) is measured using a Wright respirometer or a gas flow meter. It assesses the amount of air breathed in or out in 1 min while the individual walks on the level at a pace of 180 feet/min. It is usually 15 L/min in a healthy individual.

Maximum voluntary ventilation

Maximum voluntary ventilation (MVV) is the largest amount of air that can be breathed per minute. It is the limit of the ventilation available in reserve for exercise (**Figure 2.9**) and is about 120 L/min in a healthy individual. It can be measured in a number of ways:
- Directly using a maximal breathing test with a spirometer. The measurement is made for 15 s and the result is calculated and recorded in litres/minute. The sensitivity of a direct test using a spirometer is high but the procedure can be cumbersome and physically taxing to the patient. MVV values are therefore usually obtained indirectly
- MVV values obtained indirectly are calculated from the forced expiratory volume in 0.75 s ($FEV_{0.75}$) using the following formula:

$$MVV = FEV_{0.75} \times 40$$

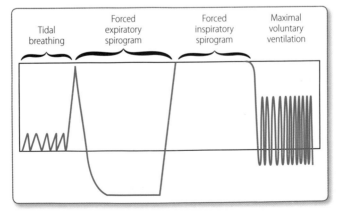

Figure 2.9 Ventilation capacities.

Ventilation indices

RMV, WV and MVV values can be compared as ratios to indicate the severity of dyspnoea in a patient. These indices include the ventilation reserve ratio and the dyspnoea index.

Ventilation reserve ratio

This is also known as the breathing reserve ratio and measures the amount of reserve in ventilation for the individual in relation to the MMV. It is calculated as:

Ventilation reserve ratio = [(MVV − RMV)/MVV] × 100.

An average MVV in a healthy individual is 120 L and the RMV is 5 L. This gives a reserve of 115 L or more than 90%. In disease RMV increases and MVV is reduced to give values of a breathing reserve ratio of 60% or less.

Dyspnoea index

This is a fairly objective grading of respiratory breathlessness. It is calculated by the ratio of walking ventilation (L/min) to maximum voluntary ventilation (L/min).

Dyspnoea index = WV/MVV.

As the average WV in a healthy individual is 15 L/min and MVV is 120 L/min, a normal dyspnoea index is 10–20%:
- < 30% indicates no dyspnoea
- > 35% mild dyspnoea
- > 45% moderate dyspnoea
- > 50% severe dyspnoea

Forced expirograph and flow–volume graphs

As mentioned above, single-breath forced spirometers report volume expired over time. Newer spirometers use flow transducers to produce graphs of flow against volume.

Forced expirograph

This reading gives the volume of gas expired over time (**Figure 2.10b**). Flow–volume inspiratory and expiratory graphs give flow rate over volumes rather than volumes against time.

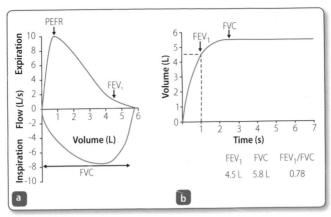

Figure 2.10 Typical flow-volume loop (a) and expirograph (b) in a healthy adult.

In this test the individual takes a full inspiration and then breathes forcibly into a spirometer with a timing device. The volume expired over a short time period, e.g. the first 0.75, 1, 2 and 3 seconds, is noted. After two practices the mean of three attempts is taken. The procedure can then be repeated after bronchodilator inhalation to record any improvement.

Flow–volume graph

Flow–volume graphs (**Figure 2.10a**) or loops have become more popular than volume–time graphs. They are particularly useful in diagnosing and monitoring mild airway obstruction when other values (such as PEFR) are only slightly abnormal.

Patients are asked to breathe normally until ready to breathe out as completely as possible to reach the point of RV. They then breathe in fully to fill up their lungs to TLC. This gives a flow–volume inspirograph. On breathing out with maximal effort, a flow–volume expirograph is

Clinical insight

- Serial measurements of FVC are taken over time to monitor improvement or decline after therapeutic interventions
- FVC is performed regularly (e.g. every 2 h) in acute presentations
- A drop in FVC of 50% of predicted (or the patient's best on admission) is an indication for intubation

produced. Forced expiration should begin rapidly and immediately on reaching the maximal inspiratory point (TLC) and continued for about 3 s or more. The procedure can then be repeated after bronchodilator inhalation. A normal example of a flow–volume graph is shown in **Figure 2.10a.**

Spirometric data

The same spirometric values (**Figure 2.11**) are obtained from the flow–volume graph as from the volume–time curve of the forced expirograph.

Forced vital capacity

The forced vital capacity (FVC) is the total amount of air (in litres) that can be forcibly blown out of the lungs in one go. It is the most common lung function test used in the hospital setting. It differs from the ordinary VC in that the breathing out after the maximal inspiration is done as fast as possible.

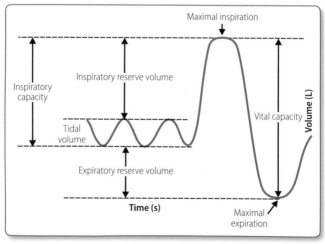

Figure 2.11 Determination of volumes and capacities from a spirometer trace.

Forced expiratory volume in 1 second

The forced expiratory volume in 1 s (FEV_1) is the amount of air (in litres) that can be forcefully blown out in one second. It is used for diagnosing airflow obstruction and grading obstruction severity as well as the response of the airway to a bronchodilator (see Chapter 4).

Normally, at least 83% of the FVC can be expired in 1 second 95% in 2 seconds and 97% in 3 seconds. Values of between 80% and 120% are usually considered to be within the normal range. Obstructive disease (asthma, chronic obstructive pulmonary disease [COPD], chronic bronchitis, emphysema) causes a reduction in FEV_1 as the increased airway resistance slows lung emptying.

FEV_1:FVC

The FEV_1:FVC ratio is a simple and important calculation to help diagnose respiratory disease. The normal FEV_1:FVC ratio is 75–80% (**Figure 2.12**). In obstructive diseases, the percentage is < 75% with near normal FVC as the blocked airway limits the speed at which exhalation can occur. Comparatively, in restrictive diseases FEV_1:FVC is > 80% but the FVC is reduced.

Maximal midexpiratory flow

Maximal midexpiratory flow (MMEF) gives a value of average flow over the midportion of the flow–volume curve, which is between 25% and 75% FVC. It is calculated by measuring the flow rate of the middle 50% of the FVC. MMEF correlates well with small airway obstruction, as it is these passages that limit flow at this midperiod of expiration.

Diffusion test

The lung's ability to transfer gases is measured as its ability to transfer carbon monoxide – the *transfer factor of the lungs for carbon monoxide* (T_LCO), also called diffusing capacity of the lung for carbon monoxide (D_LCO). This value reflects the amount of carbon monoxide taken up by the lungs in one inspiration.

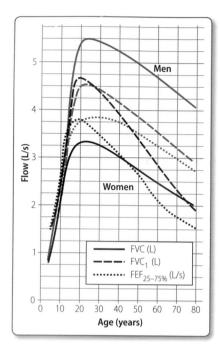

Figure 2.12 Normal values for FVC, FEV_1 and FEF_{25-75}. FEF, forced expiratory flow; FEV, forced expiratory volume; FVC, forced vital capacity.

It is therefore a measure of how well gas can cross the respiratory (alveolar–capillary) membrane.

In this procedure, the patient breathes in a test gas containing a low concentration of CO (typically 0.3%) as well as a tracer gas such as helium (10%) or methane (0.3%). After a full breath (approximating to T_LCO) of this test gas, the patient holds his or her breath for 10 seconds, then exhales smoothly but quickly. The exhaled air is collected and analysed to measure the amount of tracer gas absorbed.

The single breath method gives normal values of 15–40 mL CO/min per mmHg. The T_LCO depends on such factors as the surface area of the functioning alveoli and capillaries, and the state of permeability of the respiratory membrane across which gas diffuses. Diseases that decrease the permeability of the membrane, such as pulmonary fibrosis, will decrease $T_L CO$. Values need to be corrected for anaemia, as the haemoglobin concentration also affects the uptake of CO.

Measurements of respiratory muscle function

The mechanical work of breathing requires sufficiently functioning inspiratory muscles to lower intrathoracic pressure and draw air into the alveoli. The primary inspiratory muscles are the diaphragm and external and internal intercostal muscles. The accessory muscles used in intensive breathing include the sternocleidomastoid and scalenes.

Neuromuscular diseases exhibit a restrictive pattern on lung function testing. However, lung volume measurements are not affected by respiratory muscle weakness until there is severe impairment, and so these are not often useful where neuromuscular disease is suspected. Instead, respiratory muscle strength is assessed by looking at maximal inspiratory pressure (P_{Imax}) and maximal expiratory pressure (P_{Emax}). These tests of respiratory muscle strength are also useful when investigating an unknown cause of respiratory insufficiency:

- To obtain the P_{Imax} the patient is asked to breathe in as hard as they can and hold their breath for 2-3 seconds, with the maximum pressure of inspiration being measured at the mouthpiece
- The P_{Emax} is obtained in a similar fashion, except that patients are asked to make expiratory efforts against an occluded airway (i.e. the Valsalva manoeuvre) and the pressures are measured at total lung capacity (TLC) or functional residual capacity (FRC).

Normal values of P_{Imax} and P_{Emax} vary widely, though they are decreased in advanced neuromuscular diseases.

Tests of alveolar air distribution

These are relatively specialised tests which are used to measure the amount of air and its distribution in the alveoli. The most commonly used are nitrogen washout and single breath nitrogen meter testing.

Pulmonary nitrogen washout

This is a test to measure the amount of anatomical dead space in the lung, i.e. the volume of air that is not taking part in gaseous exchange. The patient breathes 100% O_2, 'washing out' the nitrogen in the lungs and the exhaled levels of nitrogen are then measured. Initially, only O_2 that occupied the dead space is breathed out. Gradually the percentage of nitrogen in the exhaled air increases until it plateaus at the same level as that of alveolar air.

Normally, after 7 minutes, patients have a nitrogen concentration of under 2.5%. Values above this signify an uneven distribution of alveolar air throughout the lungs, as this represents an abnormal amount of 'trapped' nitrogen due to slower emptying in some lung compartments.

Single-breath nitrogen meter test

A single-breath nitrogen meter test is used to look at the evenness of distribution of ventilation and gives an estimate of closing volume. The patient inspires a single breath of 100% O_2 and then breathes out slowly and evenly. On expiration, the nitrogen concentration rises as the dead-space gas is replaced by alveolar gas (a mixture of nitrogen and O_2). The first 750 mL of expired gas are discarded, and the nitrogen is measured in the next 500 mL expired, which is assumed to be alveolar gas. Normally the nitrogen concentration is less than 1.5% in the sample.

Alveolar oxygen tension

Alveolar O_2 tension (P_AO_2) is measured by the patient breathing through a one-way (non-re-breathing) valve with their nose closed by a nose clip. After 5 minutes the end-tidal sample of expired air is collected in a 1-L airbag for the measurement of alveolar O_2 tension. The P_AO_2 of the expired end-tidal gas sample can be analysed by either gas analyser or arterial blood gas analyser.

Disease-specific lung function tests

Bronchoprovocation testing to diagnose asthma

The diagnosis of asthma is not always easily established on the basis of history, physical examination and radiographic findings.

Furthermore, airflow obstruction is not always detectable by spirometry. Bronchoprovocation testing is useful in this clinical setting, as long as adequate resuscitation facilities are available.

A bronchoprovocation test detects bronchial hyper-responsiveness (excessive bronchoconstriction in response to various stimuli), a sign highly specific to asthma. It is important to withhold bronchodilators, within reason, before and during testing hyperresponsiveness, as they can affect the results.

Common agents include histamine or methacholine or, more recently, aerosols of hypertonic saline. Hypertonic saline produces profound bronchoconstriction in people with asthma and minimal response in normal individuals.

After breathing each requisite dose for 2 min with relaxed tidal breathing, the FEV_1 is measured at 30 and 90 s after agent nebulisation. The airway is considered hyperresponsive if FEV_1 drops by 20% or more, depending on the agent and dosage used. For example, a cut-off point for asthma diagnosis using methacholine or histamine provocation is that the concentration required to reduce FEV_1 by 20% (PC_{20}) is under 8–10 mg/ml.

Tests for exercise-induced asthma

These tests are indicated when patients have a particular subtype of asthma in which disease worsens on exercise.

A baseline FEV_1 value is obtained by spirometry. The individual is given incremental exercise until 80% of the target heart rate has been achieved. FEV_1 measurements are then recorded at 5, 10, 20 and 30 minutes. The exercise test is positive if a decline of 10% in FEV_1 is achieved. The test is negative if a 10% decline in FEV_1 is not obtained in 20–30 min.

Lung function tests in neuromuscular disease

VC can be a useful screening test in investigating respiratory muscle strength. The sensitivity of VC measurement can be increased by carrying out the test in both erect and supine positions. The VC supine is normally within 5% of the erect one and a drop of 25% is considered abnormal. In respiratory muscle weakness, a patient may display a low TLC and FVC with an increased RV and gas transfer factor.

Mouth pressures in neuromuscular disease

Mouth pressures may be abnormal in neuromuscular disease, as weakened respiratory muscles cannot generate as much intrathoracic pressure as normal.

The maximum inspiratory pressure (MIP) is the highest atmospheric pressure developed during inspiration against an occluded airway. The maximum expiratory pressure (MEP) is the highest pressure developed during expiration against an occluded airway.

The MIP and MEP can be measured using a bedside meter, while in a laboratory the transdiaphragmatic pressure (P_{DI}) is measured in sniff or twitch tests (see Chapter 6 for an explanation of these tests). The normal values for MIP and MEP given in **Table 2.5** are averages only and vary depending on age and sex.

Tilt testing

Tilt-table testing is indicated where neuromuscular disease is suspected. It measures lung capacity changes with body position. It is useful if patients complain of orthopnoea (shortness of breath when lying flat) or platypnoea (the opposite) and the cause is not obvious. It is also useful to see if the diaphragm is weak or paralysed bilaterally.

In practice, spirometry is done three times, with the patient erect (seated 90°), semi-supine (45°) and supine (180°). The VC supine is normally within 5% of the erect one and a drop of 25% is definitely abnormal. The patient is gradually laid supine while simple spirometry is performed (**Figure 2.13**). The tilt test is often combined with pulse oximetry to see the effect of position on blood O_2 saturation.

Reading	Normal value (cmH$_2$O)
Maximum inspiratory pressure	120–140
Maximum expiratory pressure	170–350

Table 2.5 Normal readings for mouth pressures.

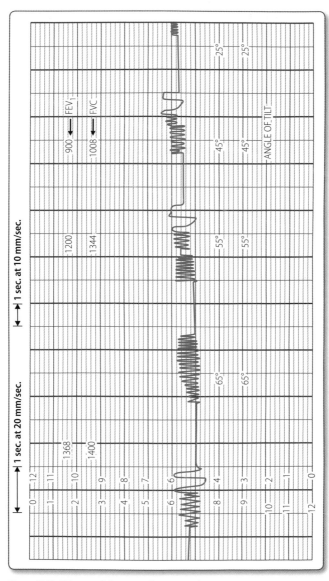

Figure 2.13 Printout of tilt test results.

Sleep studies

The clinical indications for a sleep study are given in **Table 2.6**. The two most common types of sleep study are:

- simple overnight oximetry
- full sleep study (polysomnography)

Simple overnight oximetry

For overnight oximetry studies a simple kit is used to monitor four parameters: the chest wall strap (sometimes two are used, one for the chest wall and the other for the abdomen) records chest movement, the nasal cannulae record airflow through the nose and mouth, and a finger probe records both the pulse rate and O_2 saturation (**Figure 2.14**).

Polysomnography

Polysomnography involves a range of simultaneous investigations (**Figure 2.15**):

- electroencephalogram (EEG)
- submental electromyogram (EMG)
- electro-oculogram (EOG)
- three-electrode electrocardiogram (ECG)
- thoracic movement sensors
- abdominal movement sensors
- O_2 saturation
- heart rate
- nasal airflow
- snoring
- limb movements

Loud snoring
Nocturnal arousals
Excessive daytime sleepiness
Morning headache
Decline and deterioration of intellectual function
Systemic and pulmonary hypertension
Nocturia
Unexplained polycythaemia

Table 2.6 Clinical indications for a sleep study.

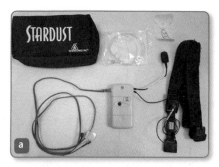

Figure 2.14 Sleep apnoea: (a) monitoring equipment; (b) monitoring in progress.

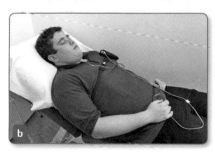

Polysomnography stages sleep and assesses respiratory airflow and effort, O_2 saturation and ECG. It identifies two states of sleep:
- Rapid eye movement (REM) sleep
- Non-rapid eye movement (NREM) sleep.

REM sleep constitutes 20–25% of total sleep and NREM sleep alternates with REM sleep throughout the night. The first REM sleep episode occurs in the second hour of sleep. Muscle atonia is characteristic of REM sleep. Rapid onset of REM sleep (< 30 min) could indicate narcolepsy, endogenous depression or drug withdrawal.

Simple overnight oximetry is less cumbersome than polysomnography and is useful as a screening device. In contrast, full polysomnography is quite invasive and expensive, and is therefore reserved for complex sleep cases.

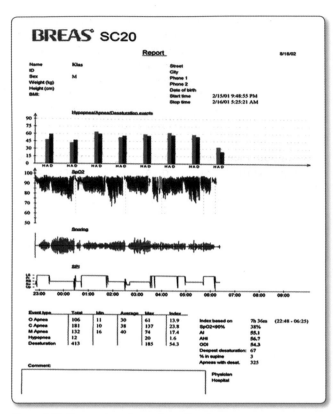

Figure 2.15 Sleep study – printout of overall results.

2.4 Exercise and fitness tests

Cardiopulmonary exercise testing

Cardiopulmonary exercise testing is an assessment of a patient's maximal cardiorespiratory function. It is useful for the evaluation of physical fitness in healthy individuals, and in assessing the level of disability in a number of cardiac and pulmonary disorders. It can be performed to assess someone for their fitness for specific tasks or for employment, as well as to determine the amount of effort that a person can safely undertake within the limits of their cardiorespiratory system.

The maximal limitations of an individual's cardiorespiratory system can be measured by O_2 uptake studies during exercise testing. The definitive measurement is the maximal O_2 uptake ($\dot{V}O_{2max}$), a measure of the body's maximum capacity to transport and use O_2 during ramped exercise testing. Indications for measuring maximal oxygen uptake ($\dot{V}O_{2max}$) are shown in **Table 2.8** (see later).

Continuous measurements of cardiac and respiratory parameters are recorded during the duration of the graded exercise (**Table 2.7**) and presented graphically (**Figure 2.16**). In some cases an ABG may be taken before and at peak exercise level.

Interpreting the results of exercise testing

Determining the anaerobic (or lactate) threshold (AT) is the most useful measure of level of fitness. The AT represents the point at which lactate is being produced by anaerobic respiration faster than the cells can clear it.

Maximal O_2 uptake is considered the best index of physical fitness and aerobic performance. Units are litres of oxygen per

Cardiac readings	Heart rate (HR) Blood pressure (BP) ECG
Respiratory readings	Tidal volume (V_T) Respiratory rate (RR) Minute ventilation ($\dot{V}_E$) Oxygen uptake ($\dot{V}O_2$) Carbon dioxide output ($\dot{V}CO_2$) Respiratory quotient (RQ)
Indices	Respiratory exchange ratio: $\dot{V}CO_2{:}\dot{V}O_2$ Oxygen uptake/heart rate (oxygen pulse) ($\dot{V}O_2$/HR) Minute ventilation/volume of oxygen uptake ($\dot{V}_E/\dot{V}O_2$) Minute ventilation/volume of carbon dioxide output ($\dot{V}_E/\dot{V}CO_2$)

Table 2.7 Values obtained in a maximal, minute-by-minute incremental cardiopulmonary exercise test

In normal individuals:
  (a) assessment of physical fitness
  (b) pre-employment assessment for specific jobs
In sports medicine:
  (a) evaluation of athletic performance
  (b) selection of training methods
  (c) sports research
In clinical medicine:
  (a) early detection of impairment of work capacity
  (b) estimate of severity of breathlessness
  (c) identification of predominance of causative factors, whether cardiac, respiratory or functional
  (d) pre- and postoperative assessment
  (e) pre- and post-therapeutic assessment
In rehabilitation programme:
  (a) work prescription appropriate to physical effort tolerance
  (b) exercise training after cardiac infarction
  (c) assessment of ability to undertake certain occupations
  (d) instituting training programmes in chronic lung disease

Table 2.8 Indications for assessing maximal aerobic capacity

minute, or a relative rate of millilitres of oxygen per minute per kilogram. Typical oxygen consumptions are higher in men than women: 30–50 ml/min per kg for (untrained) men and 30–45 ml/min per kg for (untrained) women. The term '$\dot{V}O_{2peak}$' is used when the $\dot{V}O_2$ uptake graph does not show a plateau on continued exercise but declines, showing a peak. A reduced rate of O_2 consumption at maximum attainable exercise ($\dot{V}O_{2peak}$) requires appropriate investigations to detect the cause of the disability.

MVV measures *maximum ventilatory capacity*, whereas $\dot{V}_E$ measures maximum ventilation achieved on exercise. The $\dot{V}_E$:MVV ratio is therefore a good index of ventilation reserve. A reduced $\dot{V}_E$:MVV ratio is a significant indication of exercise limitation.

The $\dot{V}_E$:$\dot{V}CO_2$ ratio is a measure of inefficient ventilation at the point AT in **Figure 2.16**. However, $P_{A-a}O_2$ (alveolar–arterial O_2 gradient) is a precise indicator of gas exchange.

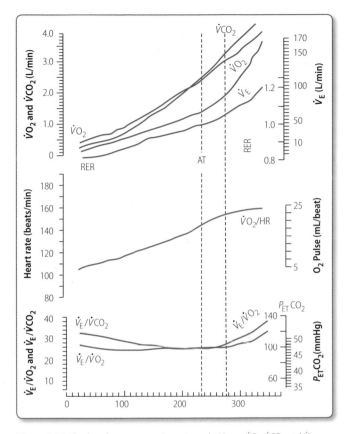

Figure 2.16 Cardiopulmonary exercise test graph. *Upper:* $\dot{V}O_2$, $\dot{V}CO_2$ and $\dot{V}_E$ values increase as work rate increases. With increased work rate during exercise testing, increase in $\dot{V}O_2$ is linear. $\dot{V}CO_2$ and $\dot{V}_E$ increase linearly with $\dot{V}O_2$ until 60% of $\dot{V}O_{2max}$, when $\dot{V}CO_2$ and $\dot{V}_E$, which remain closely linked, rise disproportionately to $\dot{V}O_2$ due to increases in lactic acid. The transition of this slope is called the anaerobic threshold (AT). The respiratory exchange ratio ($\dot{V}CO_2{:}\dot{V}O_2$) is < 1 below the AT and > 1 above the AT. *Middle, lower:* equivalent ventilation for $\dot{V}O_2$, i.e. $\dot{V}_E/\dot{V}O_2$ and ventilation. The equivalent for $\dot{V}CO_2$ is $\dot{V}_E/\dot{V}CO_2$. HR, heart rate; $P_{ET}CO_2$, end-tidal CO_2 pressure. See text for other definitions.

Six-minute walk test

This test is commonly used to assess someone's suitability for major interventions (e.g. lung transplantation) or to see if there has been an improvement after a specific therapeutic procedure. Unlike formal cardiorespiratory testing no specialised equipment is needed other than a pulse oximeter.

The patient rests for a short period and then walks along a flat surface for 6 minutes. The distance walked during this time, the presence of symptoms during the walk, and whether or not the patient was able to complete the full 6 minutes are all recorded. The results are used as an indication of qualitative respiratory function. Other baseline and post-walk measurements such as heart rate may also be recorded as an indication of fitness.

Fitness to fly

Air travel involves spending time in an environment at low atmospheric pressure. Because of the lower PO_2 at altitude, this may be poorly tolerated by patients with chronic respiratory disease. Lung function testing is often used by clinicians to assess whether such patients are fit to fly and, if they are fit, whether supplemental O_2 will be required for the trip.

Oxygen pressure at altitude

Although the fraction of inspired O_2 (F_iO_2) remains relatively constant at any altitude, the partial pressure of inspired O_2 (P_iO_2) is directly related to barometric pressure (**Table 2.9**). This, in turn, is inversely related to elevation above sea level, i.e. the higher a plane flies, the lower the barometric pressure and the lower the P_iO_2. Patients with significant lung disease can be sensitive to even relatively minor changes in P_iO_2.

Clinical scenario

The following three case scenarios show examples of maximal aerobic capacity during cardiorespiratory testing. The graphs produced from testing are shown in **Figure 2.17**.

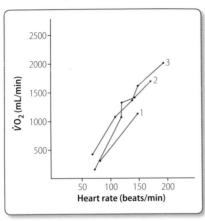

Figure 2.17 Three patterns of aerobic work capacity: (1) cardiac infarction in chronic obstructive pulmonary disease; (2) healthy untrained person; (3) trained athlete.

1. Case: a 56-year-old man who is asymptomatic but with a previous history of ischaemic heart disease and COPD.

   Test result: This man could perform on the treadmill for just 2 min at a speed of 1.7 mph at a 10° gradient. His heart rate at the peak of exercise was 144 beats/min and O_2 consumption 1144 mL/min, corresponding to an energy cost of 5.7 cal/min.

   Interpretation: His performance suggests he has severe cardiorespiratory impairment.

2. Case: a 42-year-old man who is healthy but not used to physical exercise.

   Test result: This man could perform on the treadmill for 10 min at speeds of 1.7, 3, 4 and 5 mph at a 10° gradient. He achieved a peak heart rate of 173 beats/min and O_2 consumption 1678 mL/min, corresponding to an energy cost of 8.38 cal/min.

   Interpretation: These results are consistent with a healthy untrained male.

3. Case: a 24-year-old man who is a football player with normal pulmonary function.

   Test result: His maximal aerobic capacity was 2000 mL/min. O_2 consumption was at an energy cost of 10 cal/min.

   Interpretation: This aerobic performance is consistent with him being a trained athlete.

Altitude (m)	Air pressure (mmHg)	P_iO_2 (mmHg)	P_iO_2 (kPa)
0	760	159.1	21.2
1000	674.4	141.2	18.8
2000	596.3	124.9	16.7
3000	525.8	110.1	14.7
4000	462.8	96.9	12.9
5000	405	84.8	11.3
6000	354	79.1	10.5
8000	267.8	56.1	7.5
8848	253	43.1	5.7

Table 2.9 Interrelationship of altitude, air pressure and inspired oxygen (P_iO_2).

During the flight

Most commercial airlines fly at altitudes between 22 000 feet (6700 m) and 44 000 feet (13 400 m). At these elevations the ambient barometric pressure falls from the normal 760 mmHg at sea level to between 326 and 140 mmHg, respectively. This causes a decrease in P_iO_2 with the result being the equivalent of breathing a F_iO_2 of between 8 and 3%.

Compressing ambient air is what makes commercial travel possible at these altitudes, resulting in a cabin pressure between 565 and 627 mmHg (75.3 and 83.6 kPa) at 6000–8000 feet (1829–2438 m) or an F_iO_2 equivalent to 15% and 16% at sea level.

A normal cabin environment is not only hypobaric but also effectively hypoxic.

The physiological effects of exposure to altitude

In a pressurised aeroplane cabin, breathing air at 8000 feet (2438 m) and 5000 feet (1524 m) is equivalent to breathing with F_iO_2 15.1–17.1% at sea level. In healthy individuals exposed to these conditions the P_aO_2 will be influenced by age and minute ventilation but it is likely to fall to 53–64 mmHg (7–8.5 kPa). The situation is very different in patients with chronic lung disease. At sea level such patients may already have lower P_aO_2 due to their lung disease.

In the pressurised cabin the fall in inspired O_2 pressure will lead to further fall in P_aO_2 and can result in significant

hypoxaemia during the flight. This hypoxaemia may lead to dyspnoea, increasing pulmonary hypertension and an increase in the work of breathing and cardiac workload.

For some patients, flying can be made safer by breathing supplemental O_2 during the flight. This is provided by most airlines but must be requested in advance of the flight. Airlines should be able to provide O_2 at the rate 2–4 L/min; 2 L/min is probably suitable for most patients, but those already requiring O_2 at sea level will need more. Caution is required in patients where hypoxia is their predominant respiratory drive.

Preflight assessment

All patients with chronic respiratory disease, and those with other conditions such as cardiac failure that may be worsened by hypoxia, should undergo a preflight medical assessment. Three different procedures are used to make this assessment:
- The 50-metre walk test;
- Calculating predicted hypoxia; and
- Hypoxic challenge tests.

The 50-metre walk test

Most airline medical departments favour ability to walk 50 metres without distress as a simple test for fitness to fly, though it is of little use clinically. Failure to complete the walk distress free may be an indication that in-flight O_2 is needed.

Predicting hypoxia

Several prediction equations based on a person's P_aO_2 at sea level can be used to estimate their in-flight levels of hypoxia. It can be assumed that patients with a constant S_aO_2 of 95% will not need in-flight O_2, whereas those in whom the level is < 92% will. Patients with readings of between 92% and 95% will need a further assessment. A number of different formulae can be used to predict the partial pressure of oxygen (in mmHg) for a given individual:

$P_aO_2 \text{ (alt)} = 0.410 \times P_aO_2 + 17.652$

$P_aO_2 \text{ (alt)} = 0.519 \times P_aO_2 \text{ (ground)} + 11.855 \times FEV_1 \text{ (L)} - 1.760$

$P_aO_2 \text{ (alt)} = 0.453 \times P_aO_2 \text{ (ground)} + 0.386 \times (FEV_1 \text{ % predicted}) + 2.44$

$P_aO_2 \text{ (alt)} = 22.8 - (2.74 \times \text{Altitude in 1000s of feet}) + 0.08 \times P_aO_2 \text{ (ground)}$

These formulae are useful for understanding the physiological changes at altitude but are in practice only used as a guide. Clinically, hypoxia testing (e.g. 50-metre walk test) is much more accurate.

Hypoxic challenge tests

The ideal test for assessment to fly will use a variety of methods to replicate the hypoxic environment of an aircraft cabin and record O_2 saturation for a fixed period in the simulated environment. Hypoxic challenge testing is the preflight test of choice for patients with hypercapnia.

If the P_aO_2 falls to < 50 mmHg/S_aO_2 < 85% during the hypoxic challenge, it is recommended that the patient uses supplemental O_2 throughout the flight or avoids flying altogether (**Table 2.10**). In the range 50–55 mmHg for P_aO_2, the result is borderline and some airlines may then request passengers to undergo a 50-metre walk test.

S_aO_2 (%)	P_aO_2 (mmHg) (kPa)
97	95–105 (12.6–14)
94	70–75 (9.3–10)
92	67–73 (8.9–9.5)
90	58–62 (7.7–8.3)
87	52–58 (6.9–7.7)
84	46–52 (6.1–6.9)
Guideline threshold of travellers for advising in-flight O_2 therapy	
82–84	< 50 (< 6.7)

Table 2.10 Correlations between S_aO_2 and P_aO_2.

Reproducibility of lung function testing

The reproducibility of lung function testing is important both to accurately diagnose disease and to identify patients who may be malingering or are presenting with Münchhausen's syndrome.

The following rules should be applied to all lung function tests to look for reproducibility:

- Are the two largest FVCs (forced vital capacities) within 0.2 L of each other?
- Are the two largest FEV_1 (forced expiratory volume in 1 s) values within 0.2 L of each other?

If both of these criteria are met, the test session may be concluded as being accurate. If both of these criteria are not met, testing should continue until both of them are met or a total of at least eight tests has been performed, three of which have been saved for further detailed analysis.

Figures 2.18 and **2.19** show normal flow–volume and volume–time graphs obtained from good technique, alongside examples of poor-technique graphs. The latter may be due to technical error, the patient having difficulty fully understanding the procedures involved, or malingering by the patient.

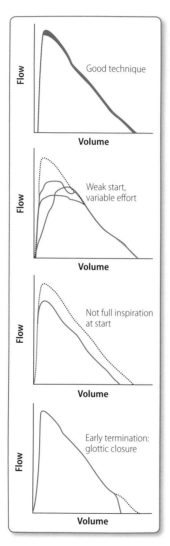

Figure 2.18 Patterns of flow–volume graphs seen with poor technique.

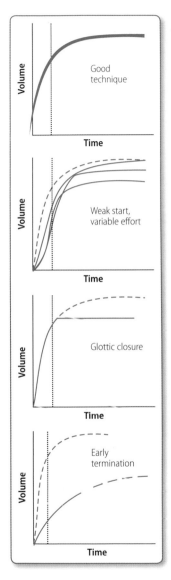

Figure 2.19 Abnormalities in volume–time graphs.

Clinical scenario

A 43-year-old woman is seen in the chest outpatient clinic with a history of asthma that is difficult to control despite her GP having tried a number of different medications. Her PEFR reading over the course of 2 weeks shows a classic diurnal variation and she is sent for formal lung function testing. Three immediate repeats show:

- FEV_1 3.2, 2.6 and 3.8 L
- FVC is equally variable
- FEV_1:FVC ratio remaining fairly constant at 60%

The PEFR recordings from home in combination with the FEV_1:FVC ratios from the lung function laboratory both suggest classic obstructive airway disease. However, the widely variable FEV_1 and FVC results suggest that there may be an element of malingering and it is important to rule this out with a detailed history as well as repeated lung function tests over a period of time, before embarking on any further management of her asthma.

Recognising abnormal results

The ability to recognise abnormal patterns in lung function and ABGs allows a rapid narrowing of the differential diagnosis. For example, an obstructive or restrictive lung spirometry pattern in a person with long-standing shortness of breath can point towards a particular type of respiratory disease. Likewise, a blood gas abnormality that can be easily identified as primarily metabolic or respiratory in nature can also help rapidly narrow down the cause of an acute illness.

3.1 Arterial blood gas abnormalities

ABGs are one of the first tests done on any critically ill patient, as they can give quick and vital information on blood oxygenation, alveolar ventilation and tissue perfusion. In interpreting ABG results, it is useful to group abnormalities as primarily a disturbance of:

- acid–base balance
- ventilation and oxygenation

Identification of critical ABG results

Important ABG changes that suggest that a patient is in a critical condition are shown in **Table 3.1**.

Acid–base disturbances

Results from an ABG can show whether there is an acidotic or alkalotic disturbance of the blood, and whether the cause of the imbalance is respiratory (i.e. related to either breathing

Guiding principle

Definitions:
Acidaemia – blood pH is < 7.35
Acidosis – the process causing acid to accumulate, usually causing acidaemia
Alkalaemia – blood pH is > 7.45
Alkalosis – the process causing alkali to accumulate, usually causing alkalaemia.
Note: the terms acidosis and alkalosis are commonly used in place of acidaemia and alkalaemia, respectively

ABG measure	Change	Indication of severity
pH	↓	Low pH indicates a level of acidosis that is damaging to tissues and organs
PCO_2	↑	May rise if patient becomes more drowsy, indicating need for assisted ventilation
PO_2	↓	May fall if patient becomes tired and cannot adequately compensate for metabolic acidosis, indicating need for assisted ventilation
Lactate	↑	High lactate indicates level of acidosis that is damaging to tissues and organs
Potassium	↑	High potassium damages to tissues (especially cardiomyocytes) and may necessitate emergency dialysis

Table 3.1 Major shifts in arterial blood gas (ABG) values which suggest the need for critical care support.

or alveolar blood diffusion) or metabolic (i.e. concerning acid and base metabolism in the blood or cells). Therefore, four patterns of acid–base disorders are classified, as shown in **Table 3.2**. These primary disorders are usually also seen with compensatory changes in blood gases, as the system attempts to retain homeostasis. In chronic disturbances of acid–base balance,

	pH	P_aCO_2 (kPa)	Standard bicarbonate (mmol/L)	Compensation
Respiratory acidosis	↓ (< 7.35)	↑ (> 6)	Normal/↑ (> 22)	Renal
Respiratory alkalosis	↑ (> 7.45)	↓ (< 4.7)	Normal/↑ (> 22)	Renal
Metabolic acidosis	↓ (< 7.35)	Normal/↓ (< 4.7)	↓ (< 20)	Respiratory
Metabolic alkalosis	↑ (> 7.45)	Normal	↑ (> 33)	Respiratory

Table 3.2 ABG values in the four different acid–base disturbances.

more compensation is usually seen, as the system has adapted to compensate to better protect the pH.

A simple algorithm in **Figure 3.1** shows how to identify quickly which acid–base disturbance is present. Some cases of mixed acid–base disturbance also occur, showing different elements of the four patterns.

The anion gap

The anion gap is a calculated estimate of the negatively charged particles in blood that are not directly measured by common blood tests. These unmeasured anions include proteins and organic acids, and the gap is based on the difference between the main measured cations (Na^+ and sometimes K^+) and anions (Cl^- and HCO_3^-). It's important to calculate and consider this value as it helps to differentiate the cause of a metabolic acidosis. A normal anion gap is 10-16 mmol/L. Metabolic acidosis with an increased anion gap is caused by excess acid, whereas a normal anion gap metabolic acidosis is from loss of base.

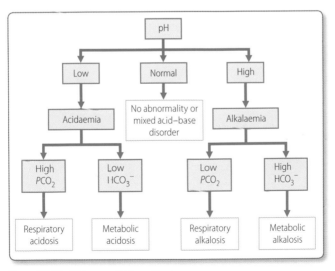

Figure 3.1 Identifying an acid–base disorder.

It can be calculated by including or, more commonly, ignoring the level of potassium (as this is usually negligible):

$$\text{Anion gap} = ([Na^+]) - ([Cl^-] + [HCO_3^-])$$
$$\text{Anion gap} = ([Na^+] + [K^+]) - ([Cl^-] + [HCO_3^-])$$

Interpreting the ABG report in five steps

The basic rules for interpreting abnormal blood gas results are shown in **Table 3.3.** Interpreting ABG results can be done in five steps:

1. pH – is the primary acid–base abnormality acidaemia (< 7.35) or alkalaemia (> 7.45)?
2. P_aCO_2 (arterial carbon dioxide tension) and bicarbonate – is it metabolic or respiratory?

Measurement	Interpretation
pH	High pH indicates alkalosis, respiratory or metabolic Low pH indicates acidosis, respiratory or metabolic
P_aO_2	High P_aO_2 may be due to hyperventilation causing a respiratory alkalosis Low P_aO_2 indicates hypoxia and supplemental O_2 may be needed
P_aCO_2	High P_aCO_2 may indicate hypoventilation, leading to a respiratory acidosis Low P_aCO_2 may be due to hyperventilation, leading to respiratory alkalosis
HCO_3^-	High bicarbonate indicates a metabolic alkalosis Low bicarbonate may be seen in metabolic acidosis (e.g. diabetic ketoacidosis)
Base excess	A more positive base excess (> +2) indicates a metabolic alkalosis A more negative base excess (< −2) indicates a metabolic acidosis
Anion gap	High anion gap indicates a loss of bicarbonate in metabolic acidosis Low anion gap may simply be due to hypoalbuminaemia

Table 3.3 Causes of changes in blood gas measurements.

3. Compensation – is it present? If not, or it is to an inappropriate level, there may be a secondary problem
4. Anion gap – this is a calculated estimate of unmeasured blood anions and is important in the context of metabolic acidosis, as it can narrow down where the acid is coming from
5. P_aO_2 – how well is the alveolar O_2 diffusing into the arteries, i.e. what is the alveolar– arterial gradient ($P_{A-a}O_2$)? Compare P_aO_2 to the inspired O_2 concentration that the patient is breathing and the P_aCO_2

Compensation

Compensatory changes seen in ABG results include increased CO_2 blow-off (hyperventilation) in metabolic acidosis and increased renal H^+ excretion in respiratory acidosis. If hypoventilation occurs there is an increase in blood CO_2 concentration and pressure, and secondary changes in the bicarbonate concentration due to renal compensation. This renal compensatory mechanism is affected by the retention of sodium ions and the excretion of hydrogen ions as ammonium chloride; the sodium is available to form more sodium bicarbonate, thus increasing the bicarbonate and attempting to maintain a HCO_3^- :P_aCO_2 20:1 ratio.

However, renal compensation is rarely complete and the pH tends to drop. In respiratory acidosis, therefore, the blood shows an increase in P_aCO_2, total CO_2 content and bicarbonate (HCO_3^-), and a decrease in pH and serum chloride concentration. In respiratory alkalosis, where a high pH results from hyperventilation, the opposite findings are observed.

Respiratory acidosis

In respiratory acidosis, there is a decrease in respiratory exchange (of O_2 with CO_2), causing retention of P_aCO_2 in the blood. This results in a high P_aCO_2 which leads to renal retention of bicarbonate in order to buffer the excess H^+. The kidneys compensate by increasing secretion of H^+ over a period of 3–5 days which results in increased plasma HCO_3^-.

Causes of respiratory acidosis are listed in **Table 3.4**.

Type of cause	Cause
Central	Drugs, e.g. morphine and sedatives Stroke Infection
Airway obstruction	Asthma Chronic obstructive pulmonary disease (COPD)
Parenchymal emphysema	Pneumoconiosis Bronchitis Acute respiratory distress syndrome Barotrauma
Neuromuscular	Poliomyelitis Kyphoscoliosis Myasthenia gravis Muscular dystrophies
Miscellaneous	Obesity Hypoventilation

Table 3.4 Causes of respiratory acidosis.

Respiratory alkalosis

Respiratory alkalosis is caused by alveolar hyperventilation, so that excessive CO_2 is exhaled and a low P_aCO_2 results. Renal compensation is by decreasing ammonium (NH_4^+) excretion, leading to a fall in HCO_3^-.

Causes of respiratory alkalosis are listed in **Table 3.5**.

Metabolic acidosis

Metabolic acidosis results from the body producing too much acid or from the kidneys failing to excrete enough. This acid accumulation causes a primary decrease in HCO_3^- as carbonic acid is produced to buffer the acid. The lungs compensate by hyperventilation, which decreases P_aCO_2 as CO_2 is blown off.

The anion gap calculation is important to differentiate the cause of a metabolic acidosis. If the anion gap is normal, this means that bicarbonate is being lost, either in the gastro-intestinal tract (e.g. diarrhoea) or by renal disease letting it leak out. A high anion gap results from increased production of

Type of cause	Cause
Central nervous system stimulation	Pain Anxiety, psychosis Fever Cerebrovascular accident Meningitis Encephalitis Trauma
Hypoxaemia or tissue hypoxia	High altitude Pneumonia Pulmonary oedema Aspiration Severe anaemia
Drugs or hormonal causes	Pregnancy Progesterone Salicylates Nikethamide
Stimulation of thoracic neural receptors	Haemothorax Flail chest Cardiac failure Pulmonary embolism
Miscellaneous	Septicaemia Mechanical hyperventilation Hepatic failure Heat exposure Recovery from metabolic acidosis

Table 3.5 Causes of respiratory alkalosis. Most mechanisms increase pH by hyperventilation and CO_2 blow-off.

organic acids (e.g. lactic acid, urate or diabetic ketoacidosis) or ingestion of large amounts of acid (e.g. aspirin overdose).

Causes of metabolic acidosis are listed in **Table 3.6**.

Metabolic alkalosis

Metabolic alkalosis is the result of an increase of HCO_3^- due to either a decreased H^+ concentration (e.g. by copious vomiting) or a direct increase in HCO_3^-. The latter can occur from bicarbonate retention, an intracellular shift of H^+ or by ingestion of

Type of metabolic acidosis	Cause
High anion gap	Lactic acidosis Ketoacidosis, e.g. diabetes, alcohol abuse, starvation Renal failure: acute and chronic. Toxins, e.g. methanol, ethylene glycol, salicylates
Normal anion gap	
Bicarbonate loss from gastrointestinal tract	Diarrhoea Extrarenal pancreatic or small bowel drainage Ureterosigmoidostomy Drugs, e.g. calcium chloride (acidifying agents), magnesium sulphate
Renal acidosis	Proximal renal tubular acidosis Distal renal tubular acidosis Tubulointerstitial disease
Drug induced	Potassium-sparing diuretics, e.g. amiloride, spironolactone Trimethoprim Pentamidine Angiotensin-converting enzyme (ACE) inhibitors Non-steroidal anti-inflammatory drugs (NSAIDs)
Others	Rapid saline infusion Loss of potential bicarbonate (i.e. anion loss in urine)

Table 3.6 Causes of metabolic acidosis.

Guiding principle

The anion gap estimates the level of serum ions that aren't measured in routine analysis because they are difficult to measure. It can be considered a measure of organic acids such as phosphate, ketones and lactate. It is calculated by subtracting the total serum anion concentration (Cl^- and HCO_3^-) from serum cations (Na^+ and K^+). In practice, potassium is often left out because it is usually negligible. Normally, the anion gap is 10–18 mmol/L.

large amounts of alkali (e.g. antacids). The lungs compensate by slower breathing (hypoventilation) to retain CO_2, showing as a rise in P_aCO_2.

Causes of metabolic alkalosis are listed in **Table 3.7**.

Mixed acid–base disturbances

Mixed acid–base disturbances occur frequently in hospitalised patients, especially

Type of cause	Cause
Acute alkali administration	For example, milk alkali syndrome
Gastrointestinal	Vomiting Nasogastric suction Villous adenoma
Renal diuretics	Hypercalcaemia Recovery from lactic acidosis/ketoacidosis Hypokalaemia
Effective extracellular volume expansion	High renin: renal artery stenosis Accelerated hypertension Aldosteronism Cushing's syndrome Steroids

Table 3.7 Causes of metabolic alkalosis.

when critically ill. This is because many patients, especially in critical condition, can have mixed pathologies affecting pH homeostasis. They can be difficult to interpret, and a good understanding of compensatory mechanisms and its proportionality is needed. Four signs that suggest a mixed acid–base disorder is present are:

1. Compensation is not occurring, or is too little or too much
2. pH is normal but P_aCO_2 or HCO_3^- is abnormal
3. P_aCO_2 and HCO_3^- are abnormal in opposite directions
4. In metabolic acidosis, the change in HCO_3^- concentration is not proportional to the change in the anion gap

One commonly seen pattern is an increased P_aCO_2 with alkaline pH. This results from an attempt to reduce the P_aCO_2 in a patient with hypercapnic respiratory failure by hyperventilation on a mechanical ventilator. Hypercapnic alkalaemia is also seen in patients with lactic acidosis or diabetic keto acidosis (DKA) who are treated with excess bicarbonate, i.e. an anion gap metabolic acidosis with metabolic alkalosis.

If P_aCO_2 or HCO_3^- is abnormal in opposite directions, so that one is raised and the other reduced, it is likely that a mixed respiratory and metabolic acid–base disorder is present. For example, combined respiratory and metabolic acidosis presents with elevated P_aCO_2 and reduced HCO_3^-. The decrease in pH is also much more than expected from the rise in P_aCO_2 values.

In combined respiratory and metabolic alkalosis, on the other hand, the P_aCO_2 is reduced and the HCO_3^- is elevated. Similarly, the pH rise is more than you would expect when looking at the fall in P_aCO_2.

Mixed respiratory and metabolic disturbances can occur in patients with chronic obstructive pulmonary disease (COPD) who are hypercapnic with respiratory acidosis and develop a metabolic alkalosis as a result of therapy with steroids and diuretics. The pH is generally near normal.

Hypoxia

Normal P_aO_2 is 10.5–13.5 kPa. Hypoxia is therefore < 10.5 kPa, and considered severe (i.e. respiratory failure) if below 8 kPa. Hypoxia and/or hypercapnia (P_aCO_2 greater than 10 kPa) may be due to one of the following mechanisms:

1. **Low inspired oxygen** (F_iO_2) at high altitude, for example
2. **Alveolar hypoventilation** is due to a reduction in ventilation at the level of the alveoli. Causes include physical defects of the alveoli, such as pneumonia, or a depressed respiratory centre, as seen in CNS disease or obesity–hypoventilation syndromes. The alveolar–arterial O_2 gradient ($P_{A-a}O_2$) is usually normal
3. **Abnormal diffusion** occurs when the respiratory membrane disrupts O_2 (and CO_2) diffusion across it, leading to an increased $P_{A-a}O_2$ gradient. Thickened, scarred basement membranes interrupt diffusion, and are seen in diseases such as pulmonary interstitial fibrosis, sarcoidosis and asbestosis. Diffusion of O_2 is affected to a greater extent than that of CO_2 because the latter diffuses at 20 times the rate
4. **Ventilation – perfusion mismatch** is when ventilation is not matching blood perfusion through the alveolar capillaries, the most common reason for hypoxia. An example is a pulmonary embolism. The ventilation–perfusion ratio ($\dot{V}/\dot{Q}$) represents the ratio between alveolar ventilation and capillary perfusion
5. **Shunts** are when blood meant for the pulmonary capillary bed bypasses it. There are various shunt mechanisms. For example, gravity exerts a physiological shunt on lung blood supply, and

a normal anatomical shunt occurs due to collateral veins (e.g. the thebesian veins draining the myocardium). A right-to-left cardiac shunt is when blood moves from the right circulation to the left due to openings between atria, ventricles or great vessels, and right heart pressure is greater than left

It is important to remember diseases can cause hypoxia or hypercapnia through one *or more* of the above mechanisms.

$\dot{V}/\dot{Q}$ ratio

Of the five causes of hypoxia, one of the most clinically important in acute situations is $\dot{V}/\dot{Q}$ mismatch. The ratio $\dot{V}/\dot{Q}$ is a measurement used to assess how well matched air and blood supply to the lungs are, as they are the main two variables determining blood O_2 concentration. It is measured with a $\dot{V}/\dot{Q}$ scan involving a gamma camera capturing subsequent images of lung ventilation and lung perfusion using inhaled and injected gamma radiation-emitting radioisotopes.

$\dot{V}/\dot{Q}$ scans are useful in localising radiographically-negative pathologies, such as pulmonary embolism.

The units

The units of the $\dot{V}/\dot{Q}$ ratio are g/L, as ventilation is recorded in grams of O_2 per minute and perfusion is presented as litres of blood per minute. Areas of lung that are underventilated relative to their blood flow have a decreased $\dot{V}/\dot{Q}$ ratio.

$\dot{V}/\dot{Q}$ mismatch

A number of clinical conditions disturb the $\dot{V}/\dot{Q}$ ratio, including atelectasis, aspiration pneumonia and pulmonary emboli. These conditions can all alter the interface between air and blood and hence cause a mismatch in the $\dot{V}/\dot{Q}$ ratio in a part of the lung that is damaged. The $P_{A-a}O_2$ is usually significantly widened in these patients, and they respond poorly to supplemental O_2.

> ## Guiding principle
>
> $\dot{V}/\dot{Q}$ ratio:
> - Is increased where ventilation is greater than perfusion, which causes decreased P_aO_2 and increased P_aCO_2
> - Is decreased where perfusion is greater than ventilation, which leads to decreased P_aO_2 (and rarely decreased P_aCO_2)
> - **Shunt** = $\dot{V}/\dot{Q}$ of 0 = area with no ventilation
> - **Dead space** = $\dot{V}/\dot{Q}$ of ~infinity = area with no perfusion

For the purposes of management, it is useful to categorise patients by three patterns of $\dot{V}/\dot{Q}$ mismatch:

1. **A mismatch of $\dot{V}$ and $\dot{Q}$ but with normal respiratory control** occurs with, for example, pneumonia, pulmonary embolus and moderate asthma. Normal respiratory control means that their respiratory drive is sensitive to both P_aO_2 and P_aCO_2, and they can therefore be given O_2 at any concentration necessary to achieve satisfactory P_aO_2.

2. **Marked mismatch of $\dot{V}$ and $\dot{Q}$ with significant right-to-left shunting** is seen in patients with, for example, pulmonary oedema and acute respiratory distress syndrome. They are difficult to oxygenate by increasing F_iO_2 alone and require ventilatory support to improve O_2 transfer.

3. **Mismatch of $\dot{V}$ and $\dot{Q}$, with dysfunction of respiratory control** in patients with ventilatory failure, e.g. alveolar hypoventilation and COPD with raised P_aCO_2. They are given controlled administration of O_2 or ventilatory support when required. In respiratory diseases with obstructive defects, the cause of arterial hypoxia is a low $\dot{V}/\dot{Q}$, due to either increased resistance as in asthma and bronchitis or increased compliance as in emphysema.

Respiratory failure

Most of the causes of hypoxia discussed above, if sustained and severe enough, can lead to respiratory failure (a P_aO_2 below 8 kPa). Disturbed pulmonary gas exchange leads to low P_aO_2 with or without raised P_aCO_2. The mechanisms leading to respiratory failure are similar to those leading to hypoxia (discussed above).

Respiratory failure is due to one of three mechanisms, each presenting different patterns on ABGs (**Table 3.8**):

- Inadequate *ventilation* of gases into alveoli
- Inadequate *diffusion* of gases across the respiratory membrane
- Inadequate blood *perfusion*

Type I and II respiratory failure

Due to important differences in how they respond to O_2 treatment, patients are also divided into type I and type II

Type of failure	Causes
Ventilatory	Upper airway pathology, e.g. obstructive sleep apnoea, foreign body aspiration Lower airway pathology, e.g. cancers, obstructive airway disease Muscle pathology, e.g. myopathy, trauma Neurological disease, e.g. motor neuron disease, central respiratory depressant drugs
Diffusion	Pleural causes, e.g. pneumothorax, pleural effusions Parenchymal causes, e.g. bronchiectasis, obstructive airway disease
Perfusion	Pulmonary embolism Intracardiac shunting

Table 3.8 Causes of respiratory failure.

respiratory failure (**Table 3.9**). Type I is hypoxia ($P_aO_2 < 8$ kPa) with a normal/low P_aCO_2 and is caused by $\dot{V}/\dot{Q}$ mismatch. Type II is hypoxia and hypercapnia ($P_aCO_2 > 6.0$ kPa) and is caused by hypoventilation with or without a $\dot{V}/\dot{Q}$ mismatch. Treatment in either case is O_2 and respiratory support, but caution is essential in type II respiratory failure, as patient's may develop dangerously high hypercapnia because of their dependency on hypoxic respiratory drive.

Ventilatory failure

If the $P_{A-a}O_2$ is near normal (1.3–2.6 kPa), isolated ventilatory failure is present. There is often some additional abnormality in the airways or the lungs to account for an increased $P_{A-a}O_2$. However, in ventilatory failure, hypoxaemia is usually easily corrected either by providing adequate alveolar ventilation mechanically or by a small increase in the F_iO_2. Any form of ventilatory failure can be type I or type II.

Diffusion failure

This is usually caused by pleural or parenchymal disease and represents a failure of gases to diffuse across the alveoli.

Type of failure	ABG results	Causes	Response to oxygen therapy
Type I	• P_aO_2 low (< 8.0 kPa) • P_aCO_2 normal or low • $P_{A-a}O_2$ increased	Asthma, pneumonia and pulmonary embolism	Usually fine
Type II	• PaO_2 decreased (< 8.0 kPa) • P_aCO_2 increased (> 6.0 kPa) • $P_{A-a}O_2$ normal • pH decreased	**Pulmonary:** asthma, COPD, pneumonia, fibrosis **Neuromuscular:** myasthenia gravis, Guillain–Barré syndrome, poliomyelitis, Cervical spine injury **Reduced respiratory drive:** sedatives, CNS disease **Anatomical:** kyphoscoliosis	At risk of hypercapnia due to loss of central respiratory drive. Give controlled O_2 and monitor ABGs

Table 3.9 Types of respiratory failure.

Clinical insight

Monitoring ABGs in respiratory failure:

• Type I respiratory failure, e.g. asthma: one initial ABG, after which pulse oximetry is sufficient for monitoring blood oxygen levels
• Type II respiratory failure, e.g. COPD: ABGs are used regularly to monitor PaO_2, as it can rapidly decline. $PaCO_2$ also needs to be monitored in these patients, as their hypercapnic central respiratory drive is often diminished

Perfusion defects

Unlike in ventilatory failure, a $\dot{V}/\dot{Q}$ mismatch leads to an increase in the $P_{A-a}O_2$. This mechanism is a frequent cause of hypoxaemia when there is severe, overwhelming and often acute lung disease.

Mismatching of alveolar ventilation and pulmonary blood flow may be so marked that areas of the lungs may have a $\dot{V}/\dot{Q}$ ratio of nearly zero, a situation tantamount to a shunt, i.e. there is an increased amount of right-to-left intrapulmonary shunting. This usually occurs in acute lung injury when the lung volume has decreased acutely with a decrease in compliance. Hypoxaemia due to shunting is frequently severe and usually resistant to an increase in F_iO_2.

3.2 Lung function testing abnormalities

Pulmonary function is only an indication of how lungs are functioning and provides no specific pathological diagnosis. They therefore must be considered in context of the history, examination and other investigations. A simple algorithm can be used to quickly identify the main type of lung defect, and to suggest further investigations needed (**Figure 3.2**).

Understanding the basic abnormalities seen in simple spirometry testing can be helpful in diagnosing respiratory, cardiac, metabolic and neurological diseases. Aside from the specific changes associated with different diseases (which are

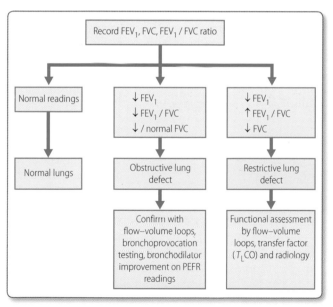

Figure 3.2 Identifying a lung defect using spirometry in a clinical context.

described in detail in the relevant chapters), an understanding of abnormalities of diffusion and of gas exchange will help interpret changes seen in spirometry and help diagnose the cause.

A normal result is relative to age, gender and height. Normal ranges are the outcome of large population studies, though different studies give different ranges.

Guiding principle

Static lung function measurements alone are not as helpful as serial measurements taken over time to indicate improvement or decline after therapeutic interventions.

Types of ventilatory defects

The main patterns of flow–volume loops seen in different diseases are shown in **Figure 3.3** and described in **Table 3.10**. They can generally be grouped into obstructive, restrictive or mixed patterns.

Obstructive ventilatory defects

An obstructive abnormality represents a reduction in maximum airflow out of the lungs that is disproportionate to the maximal volume (i.e. the vital capacity, VC). This is due to a narrowing airway on exhalation, measured as a reduced FEV_1/VC ratio. Obstruction is defined as an FEV_1/FVC ratio of < 0.70. Changes in the flow–volume loop seen in obstructive lung defects are shown in **Figure 3.4a** and a typical forced expirograph is shown in **Figure 3.4b**.

Common obstructive lung diseases include:
- asthma
- bronchitis
- COPD

Restrictive ventilatory defects

In restrictive diseases, VC is reduced to below 80% of expected. FEV_1 and FVC are reduced proportionately, and this gives a normal FEV_1/FVC ratio. There is also a reduction in the diffusion capacity of the lung and usually a low P_aCO_2. Most cases involve pulmonary fibrosis. The changes in the

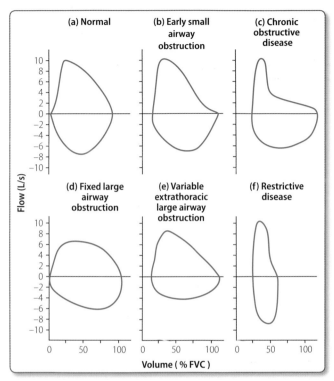

Figure 3.3 The main changes seen in the flow–volume loop.

flow–volume loop seen in restrictive lung defects are summarised in **Figure 3.5**.

Common restrictive lung diseases include:

- interstitial lung disease
- infectious inflammation, e.g. histoplasmosis
- neuromuscular diseases
- chest wall deformities

Mixed ventilatory defects

A mixed ventilatory defect shows evidence of both obstruction and restriction, so that both the FEV_1/FVC ratio and TLC

Disease	Changes seen in flow–volume loop
Obstructive lung disease, e.g. asthma or COPD	Flow rate low in relation to lung volume; reversibility may be seen after bronchodilator, giving more normal flow–volume loop
Fixed large airway obstruction, e.g. goitre	Plateau at low flows in both the expiratory and inspiratory phases
Variable extrathoracic large airway obstruction, e.g. vocal cord paralysis	Plateau at inspiratory phase but expiratory pattern is normal
Restrictive disease	Total volume expired and maximum flow rate reduced. Flow high in late part of expiration, giving characteristic flow–volume loop seen in disease

Table 3.10 Flow–volume loop patterns in disease.

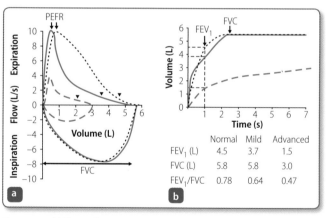

Figure 3.4 (a) Flow-volume graphs and (b) forced expirographs showing normal (dashed black), mild (blue) and severe (dashed blue) obstructive lung defects. FEV_1, forced expiratory volume in 1 second (arrowheads); FVC, forced vital capacity; PEFR, peak expiratory flow rate.

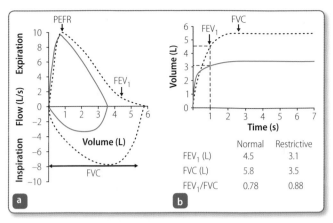

Figure 3.5 (a) Flow–volume graph and (b) forced expirograph showing a restrictive lung defect (blue line). FEV, forced expiratory volume; FVC, forced vital capacity; PEFR, peak expiratory flow rate.

are below 80% of their predicted values. Consequently, both curvilinear (i.e. obstructive) and miniature (i.e. restrictive) patterns are seen on flow–volume loops.

T_LCO

T_LCO is useful to differentiate restrictive defects. It is lowered in any disease that decreases the amount of functioning respiratory membrane, such as emphysema, pulmonary embolism or interstitial fibrosis. A normal value indicates that the cause of restriction is probably outside the lungs, e.g. a chest wall deformity or obesity.

Lung diseases

Lung diseases are associated with abnormalities in lung function and arterial blood gas (ABG) status. The different conditions can be grouped according to where they affect the respiratory tract from the airways to the parenchyma, and from the blood vessels through to the pleura and chest wall.

Patterns of lung function can be used to diagnose disease with a high degree of certainty in some cases, for example:

- A reversible obstructive pattern in a person with a history suggestive of asthma helps confirm the diagnosis
- A non-reversible obstructive pattern in a person with a similar clinical picture but a long history of smoking points towards a diagnosis of chronic obstructive pulmonary disease (COPD)

Lung function testing can also be used to assess or monitor the severity of lung disease in the short or long term. For example, a gradual reduction over a period of months in the forced expiratory volume in 1 s (FEV_1) is evidence of worsening emphysema.

ABGs can be used to create an immediate picture of an acute situation, e.g. a low partial pressure of oxygen (PO_2) despite maximal oxygen via a facemask may indicate that a patient with asthma needs ventilatory support.

A number of respiratory disorders have associated cardiac abnormalities (e.g. cor pulmonale in COPD) that need to be considered when assessing the respiratory status.

4.1 Airway disease

Obstructive diseases are characterised by ventilatory (i.e. airway) dysfunction. A common application of spirometry in obstructive disease is dynamic testing of ventilatory capacity, e.g. FEV_1, FEV_1 as the percentage of the forced vital capacity (% FVC), maximum voluntary ventilation (MVV), pulmonary flow rate (PFR) and maximum midexpiratory flow (MMEF). By seeing the effect of medications such as bronchodilators and steroids on these values, disease progress can be monitored and management can be refined.

Lung function tests are useful if done serially to study the progress of airway disease and re-evaluate prognosis. This is very important in COPD management, for example.

Advanced obstructive diseases can also involve disturbances of gas exchange, diffusion and perfusion so that monitoring of blood gases is important in these cases.

Asthma

Asthma is an increased hyperresponsiveness of the bronchial tract characterised by widespread narrowing of the airways on exposure to multiple stimuli, which is reversible either spontaneously or by drug therapy.

> ### Clinical insight
>
> Cough, especially at night, can be a hallmark feature of asthma. Other causes of chronic cough include gastro-oesophageal reflux and chronic irritable cough syndrome.

> ### Guiding principle
>
> Airflow obstruction in asthma is often rapidly and completely reversible by an adequate dose of bronchodilator.

The main pathogenic feature of asthma is non-specific hyperirritability of the bronchial tract that develops as a result of active airway inflammation. The airways are oedematous with infiltration by eosinophilia, neutrophils, lymphocytes and mast cells, as well as increased vascularity and thickening of the basement membrane. The cells release mediators that produce an inflammatory reaction involving bronchoconstriction, vascular congestion and oedema.

Changes in lung function

The following lung function measures are reduced during asthma attacks, and return virtually to normal after bronchodilators are administered:

- FEV_1
- FEV_1 as % FVC

- MVV
- MMEF
- peak expiratory flow rate (PEFR)

Detailed lung function testing can determine the exact subtype of asthma:

- **Classic asthma** shows a reversible obstructive lung disease
- **Occupational asthma** shows a reduced PEFR at work which improves after long periods away from work, e.g. on holiday
- **Exercise-induced asthma** shows a decline in FEV_1 on exercise.

As with emphysema, some reduction in vital capacity (VC), increase in residual volume (RV) and rise in the ratio RV/total lung capacity (TLC) may occur, but these changes may not be significant.

PEFR is also often reduced during asymptomatic periods (**Figure 4.1**), but a single reading cannot be used to diagnose disease. Multiple readings may show a classic diurnal variation pattern in which PEFR readings rise and fall during the course of a day (**Figure 4.2**). Improved peak flow rates can be observed when occupational asthma sufferers are absent from the workplace for an extended period of time.

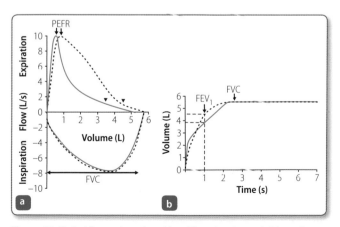

Figure 4.1 Typical flow–volume loop (a) and forced expirograph (b) seen in a person with asthma (blue line); dashed black line = normal. PEFR, peak expiratory Flow rate; FEV_1, forced expiratory volume in 1 second (arrowheads).

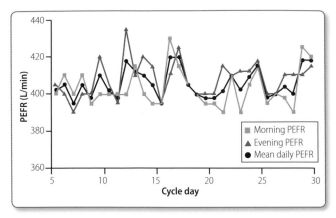

Figure 4.2 Diurnal variation in asthma. PEFR, peak expiratory flow rate.

The asthmatic flow–volume loop seen in simple spirometry shows a volume-dependent collapse , usually with a normal VC. VC may be reduced due to mucus plugging and/or trapping. T_LCO is usually normal. As with a PEFR, a single flow–volume loop is difficult to interpret by itself. Repeated readings will show a consistent picture of airflow obstruction, along with evidence of reversibility with an increase in FEV_1 after bronchodilator use (**Figure 4.3**).

Changes in ABGs

ABG testing in asthma is often normal when patients are well. In those with a mild exacerbation there may be hyperventilation, leading to a high PO_2, low PCO_2 and respiratory alkalosis (**Table 4.1**). During severe asthma attacks hypoxia, hypercapnia, respiratory acidosis and increased levels of lactate can occur (**Table 4.2**).

Guiding principle

ABGs are not usually tested in moderate exacerbations of asthma, but they can be useful for a rapid assessment of severity and the potential need for assisted ventilation.

Other tests in asthma

The diagnosis of asthma is not always clearly established on the basis of history, physical

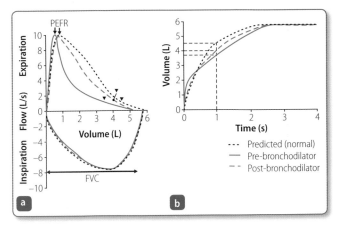

Figure 4.3 Flow–volume graph (a) and forced expirograph (b) showing obstructive ventilatory defect with reversibility after bronchodilator use. FVC, forced vital capacity; PEFR, peak expiratory flow rate.

examination and radiographic findings. Other tests, such as the bronchoprovocation test may be required (see page 48). Tests for exercise-induced asthma are described on page 49.

Chronic obstructive pulmonary disease

The term 'COPD' encompasses a spectrum of disorders, the most important of which are:
- bronchitis
- emphysema

ABG measure	Level	Change
pH	7.39	No change
PCO_2 (kPa)	4.8	No change
PO_2 (kPa)	9.2	↓
HCO_3^- (mmol/L)	23.1	No change
Lactate (mmol/L)	0.6	No change

Table 4.1 Arterial blood gases in a mild asthma attack.

ABG measure	Level	Change
pH	7.29	↓
PCO_2 (kPa)	7.8	↑↑
PO_2 (kPa)	6.2	↓↓
HCO_3^- (mmol/L)	22.7	No change
Lactate (mmol/L)	4.3	↑

Table 4.2 Arterial blood gases in a severe asthma attack.

In most patients with COPD, emphysema and chronic bronchitis are concurrent.

Emphysema

This is a progressive disease in which permanent abnormal enlargement of the airspaces distal to the terminal respiratory bronchiole is accompanied by destructive changes in the alveolar walls, with consequent loss of surface area. The resulting difficulty in expelling air and the poor distribution of gases throughout the lungs are responsible for the dyspnoea that is the main presenting feature of emphysema.

Chronic bronchitis

In chronic bronchitis, the lining of the bronchi is constantly inflamed and large volumes of thick mucus are secreted, making it hard to breathe. Chronic productive cough is the main presenting feature.

Important causes of COPD

Most cases of COPD are directly linked to long-term smoking. The long-term effects of smoking appear on lung function tests as a decline in FEV, proportional to amount of smoking, and are partially reversible

Clinical insight

Lung transplantation criteria for patients with COPD vary worldwide but in general patients must have:

- end-stage COPD
- no significant comorbidities
- weight within an acceptable range
- ceased smoking

There is usually no upper age limit for lung transplantation but the paucity of donors often dictates an age limit of 60 years.

on smoking cessation (**Figure 4.4**). The level of smoking-related damage is measured in pack-years.

In some adults, severe COPD results from an inherited lack of functioning α_1-antitrypsin, an enzyme involved in lung protection. Basic spirometry cannot determine this; it requires metabolic testing of enzyme levels for confirmation. Cumulative damage leads to symptomatic lung disease between the ages of 20 and 50 years. Smoking cessation advice should be strongly given to such patients because tobacco smoke accelerates development of emphysema.

> ## Clinical insight
>
> One pack-year is calculated as a person smoking 20 cigarettes a day for 1 year. For example, a person smoking 10 cigarettes a day for 10 years will have a 5 pack-year history

Changes in lung function

Airway obstruction is a very prominent and characteristic aspect of emphysema. As with asthma the airflow obstruction is measured by FEV_1 as % FVC, MVV, MMEF and PFR, all of which

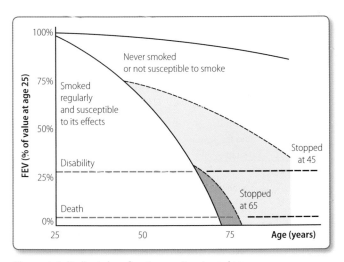

Figure 4.4 Decline in lung function over time in smokers.

Clinical insight

Positive airway pressure is used to treat COPD, heart failure and sleep apnoea:

- **CPAP** (continuous positive airway pressure) delivers a continuous pressure of air and is more useful in heart failure or as a form of ventilation in intensive care
- **BiPAP** (bilevel positive airway pressure) provides an inspiratory pressure and an expiratory pressure, and is more useful in patients with COPD and type II respiratory failure

are reduced in COPD. The important feature is that airway obstruction is irreversible in emphysema, therefore values do not generally improve after bronchodilator use. The physiological disturbance of emphysema differs from asthma by increased RV and the ratio RV/TLC. The RV/TLC measurement is vital and is used extensively in diagnosing emphysema and predicting its course.

The typical changes seen in COPD involve a prolonged expiratory time and a pressure-dependent collapse in the expiratory phase as seen in basic spirometry (**Figure 4.5**). The VC may be normal or increased due to air trapping. The transfer

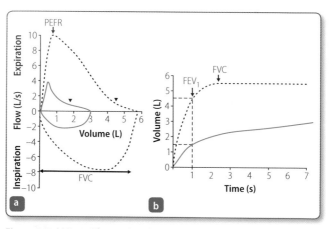

Figure 4.5 (a) Typical flow–volume loop and (b) forced expirograph in chronic obstructive pulmonary disease (solid blue line), dashed black line = normal. FEV_1, forced expiratory volume in 1 second (arrowheads); FVC, forced vital capacity; PEFR, peak expiratory flow rate.

factor $T_L CO$ may be reduced in severe disease. Unlike asthma, in COPD there are no significant changes in lung function following the administration of bronchodilators.

Changes in ABGs

COPD is associated with ventilation–perfusion disturbances due to increased capillary blood flow (perfusion) to underventilated alveoli. Measurable impairment of diffusion is found only when there is gross anatomical loss of alveolar surface area by alveolar destruction. Ultimately ventilatory disturbance results in alveolar hypoventilation, CO_2 retention, hypoxaemia and respiratory acidosis.

Acute exacerbations of COPD

ABG changes typical of mild and severe acute exacerbations of COPD are shown in **Tables 4.3** and **4.4**. Mild exacerbations often just exhibit mild hypoxaemia. Severe exacerbations

ABG measure	Level	Change
pH	7.38	No change
PCO_2 (kPa)	4.8	No change
PO_2 (kPa)	8.2	↓
HCO_3^- (mmol/L)	23.6	No change
Lactate (mmol/L)	0.8	No change

Table 4.3 Arterial blood gases in a mild COPD exacerbation.

ABG measure	Level	Change
pH	7.22	↓↓
PCO_2 (kPa)	13.8	↑↑↑
PO_2 (kPa)	3.2	↓↓↓
HCO_3^- (mmol/L)	25.7	No change
Lactate (mmol/L)	3.1	↑

Table 4.4 Arterial blood gases in a severe COPD exacerbation.

Clinical scenario

A 74-year-old woman is admitted to A&E in a drowsy state. She is a heavy smoker with a history of COPD. Her ABG on room air shows:

- pH 7.12
- PCO_2 14.3 kPa
- PO_2 8.2 kPa.

The blood gas and clinical pictures are consistent with severe respiratory acidosis and type II respiratory failure in a patient with known COPD. This acute exacerbation has resulted in a very high PCO_2 and low PO_2 and she is unable to physiologically maintain adequate ventilation. The immediate goal is to stabilise her blood gases using assisted ventilation. This may be in the form of BiPAP or she may need formal intubation and ventilation. In such a case it is important to assess her premorbid state to ensure that she is an appropriate candidate for intensive care management (see Chapter 6).

Guiding principle

Serial lung function measurements in chronic diseases are more useful than investigations in the acute phase.

commonly present with severe hypoxaemia, respiratory acidosis and lactic acidosis. Early lactate production on exercise is associated with COPD, probably due to decreased aerobic capacity of muscle fibres. Patients with acute exacerbation may need extra O_2 to help improve their oxygenation. In oxygenating these patients, there is a risk of hypercapnia due to their dependence on hypoxic respiratory drive. Type II respiratory failure and necrosis can result. In this situation assisted ventilation such as bilevel positive airway pressure (BIPAP) may be needed, but this may simply be an adjunct to formal ventilation.

Chronic bronchitis

The most important complication of chronic bronchitis is respiratory obstruction giving rise to disabling breathlessness. This is due to underlying, permanent structural changes, but almost always there is also a reversible or asthmatic element. The same set of tests used in asthma and emphysema are used to measure the obstructive defect of chronic bronchitis with similar results.

Bronchiectasis

This is an abnormal and permanent dilatation of the bronchi, either segmental or widespread in distribution. This is associated with chronic recurrent infection of the bronchiectatic area and expectoration collected there. Bronchiectasis

Log-in to get the most from Library Search using your Keele IT username and password.

Guest	★ e-Shelf	My Account	Sign in
A-Z	Citation Linker	Subject Resources	Help

Login type:

    Keele staff and students

    NHS and other users

Cancel

Physical items are indicated by **Locations** – make a note of the shelfmark to find the item on the shelves.

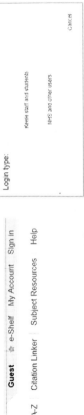

History
Athanasios Paliouras Editor
1998 3rd ed.
Book

● **Available at Campus Library Campus library (DF901 .M3P2)**

Keele University

Locations   Details   Virtual Bookshelf

Request Options: Request

Location	Campus Library . Campus library DF901 .M3P2
Availability:	(1 copy, 1 available, 0 requests)

Barcode	Type	Loan length
50968556	Book	Sessional Lo

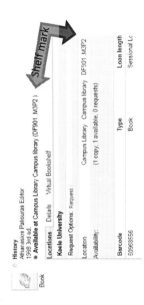

Shelf mark

Online then clicking **Books** as the resource type.

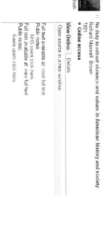

Show only

Available in the Library (3,198)
Full Text Online (419)

Refine My Results

Resource Type
Books (3,672)
Journals (708)
Audio Visual (30)
dissertations (4)
Scores (2)
More options ∨

Refine My Results

Resource Type
Books (260)
Journals (200)
More options ∨

Book

No duty to retreat: violence and values in American history and society
Richard Maxwell Brown
1991

• **Online access**

View Online | Details

Open source in a new window

Full text available at: view full text
Public note:
NPG users click here.
Full text available at: view full text
Public note:
Keele users click here

Online access and **View Online** indicate it is an electronic item. Click the **View Full Text** option for "Keele users" and you'll be taken into the e-book.

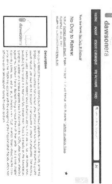

Multiple editions of an item are grouped.

Multiple Versions

A history of the world in 10 1/2 chapters
Julian, Barnes
Multiple versions found
To view, click on the title or the link to the right

Electronic and digital items are indicated by **View Online** – select the database you want to use to access the resource.

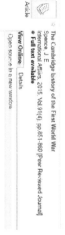

Article

Open source in a new window

The Cambridge history of the First World War
Spence, J. E.
International Affairs, 2015, Vol.91(4) pp.851-860 [Peer Reviewed Journal]
• **Full text available**

View Online   Details

Full text available at: Wiley Online Library 2015 Full Collection
Available from 1998 volume: 74 issue: 1
Full text available at: EBSCOhost Academic Search Complete
Available from 1975
Most recent 1 year(s) not available
Full text available at: EBSCOhost Business Source Complete
Available from 1975
Most recent 1 year(s) not available

2 Examples for Everything

Refined by   List of Versions   ×

A history of the world in 10 1/2 chapters
Julian, Barnes
2009
• **Available at** Campus Library Campus library (PR6052 A75B4)

Locations   Virtual Bookshelf

Book

A history of the world in 10 1/2 chapters
Julian, Barnes
1990
• **Available at** Campus Library Campus library (PR6052 A75B44)

Locations   Details   Virtual Bookshelf

Book

2 Results for Everything

E-books can be found by using the filters and clicking **Full Text**

University Hospitals
of North Midlands

NHS

NHS Trust

Library**Search**

What am I searching?

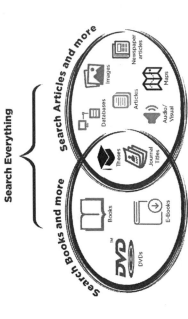

Search Everything

search Books and more

search Articles and more

Use **Search Books and More** to find "physical" items in the Library collection and e-books.

Use **Search Articles and More** to find journal articles

generally shows airflow obstruction due to either the primary pathology of bronchiectasis or any associated COPD (**Figure 4.6**).

In patients with extensive and advanced bronchiectasis, basic spirometry shows:
- A marked reduction in VC
- Increased RV
- TLC that is normal or slightly decreased

Pulmonary compliance is usually diminished and airway obstruction is present in some patients. Typically, only mild hypoxaemia is seen **Table 4.5**.

Lung function tests in patients with extensive and advanced bronchiectasis show a marked reduction in VC with increased RV, similar to the results shown in **Figure 4.5** from a patient with COPD. TLC may be normal or slightly decreased. Pulmonary compliance is usually diminished and airway obstruction is

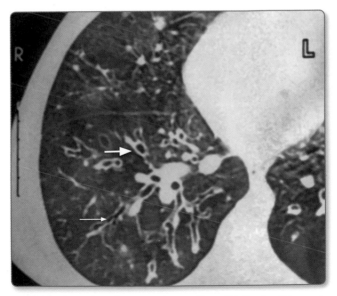

Figure 4.6 Varicose bronchiectasis with areas of bronchial dilatation (thin arrow) and wall thickening (thick arrow).

ABG measure	Level	Change
pH	7.41	No change
PCO_2 (kPa)	5.2	No change
PO_2 (kPa)	9.1	↓
HCO_3^- (mmol/L)	24.9	No change
Lactate (mmol/L)	0.8	No change

Table 4.5 Arterial blood gases in severe bronchiectasis.

present in some patients. Typically, only mild hypoxaemia is seen (**Table 4.5**).

Cystic fibrosis

In cystic fibrosis, the pathology and results of lung function tests are similar to bronchiectasis. In addition, there is lung fibrosis and segmental collapse due to significant mucus production (**Figure 4.7**). Lung function often shows an obstructive pattern (see **Figure 4.5**) with a reduced FEV_1 as well as reduced FEV_1/FVC ratio. VC may be reduced and there may

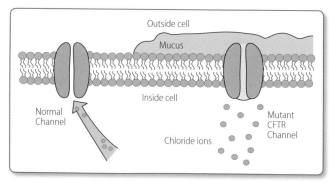

Figure 4.7 In cystic fibrosis, a normal functioning cystic fibrosis transmembrane regulator (CFTR) protein channel moves chloride ions to the outside of the cell, whereas a mutant CFTR channel does not, causing sticky mucus to build up on the outside of the cell.

be the appearance of a mixed obstructive/restrictive defect. $T_L CO$ is reduced.

ABG changes in early and severe disease are similar to those seen in bronchiectasis, with mild hypoxaemia (see **Table 4.5**). Lung function is also similar to that seen in bronchiectasis (see **Figure 4.6**).

Sleep apnoea

Obstructive sleep apnoea/hypopnoea syndrome (OSAHS) is defined as frequent episodes of apnoea and hypopnoea during sleep, with symptoms of impaired quality of life due to excessive daytime sleepiness and increased risk of sudden death during sleep. The diagnosis of OSAHS is made on the basis of:

- A suggestive clinical history,
- High Epworth Sleepiness Score (determined using a patient questionnaire) and
- A positive sleep study as determined by the level of apnoea recorded.

An episode of apnoea is defined as a complete cessation of breathing for at least 10 s with a corresponding desaturation by 3%. A hypopnoeic episode is when the amplitude of breathing measured overnight is reduced by half. These two events are used to calculate the apnoea/hypopnoea index (AHI), which is the total number of events per hour. An AHI > 5 is considered pathological. An AHI of 6–15 is interpreted as mild, 16–30 as moderate and > 30 as severe disease.

There are three types of sleep disorder:

1. **Obstructive sleep apnoea**, in which airflow at the nose and mouth is absent or reduced despite continuous respiratory effort
2. **Central sleep apnoea**, in which both the airflow and respiratory effort are absent (**Figure 4.8**)

Clinical insight

Patients diagnosed with sleep apnoea should be advised to contact the regulatory driving authority (the Driver and Vehicle Licensing Agency (DVLA) in the UK) and if they fall asleep while driving they should be told that they cannot drive until they have received appropriate treatment and their daytime sleepiness has reduced.

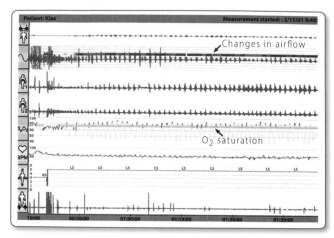

Figure 4.8 Sleep studies: an example of a 10-minute report.

3. **Mixed sleep apnoea,** in which there are both central and obstructive events

   Simple sleep studies and full sleep studies (polysomnography) are described in Chapter 2.

   The characteristic sleep study trace shows a flat line (apnoeic) or an amplitude of the airflow reduced by half (hypopnoeic). The chest wall movement may be increased in an obstructive episode or decreased in central apnoea. There is an increase in heart rate with a corresponding drop in O_2 saturations.

4.2 Parenchymal disease

Pneumonia (Table 4.6)

Lung function testing is not routinely carried out in cases of pneumonia where there is a high clinical suspicion of diagnosis. In some cases, such as in bronchiolitis obliterans organising pneumonia (BOOP), a chronic sequela of pneumonia, basic spirometry may be used to monitor the long-term response to treatment. In such cases the flow–volume loop may be similar to that seen in restrictive disease, i.e. reduced FEV$_1$ and FVC, with a normal FEV$_1$/FVC ratio (**Figure 4.9**).

Interstitial lung diseases

Interstitial lung disease is a group of diseases of various known and unknown aetiologies grouped together because they have many common clinical manifestations, e.g. dry persistent cough and persistent progressive breathlessness on exertion,

ABG measure	Level	Change
pH	7.19	↓↓↓
PCO_2 (kPa)	8.2	↑↑
PO_2 (kPa)	6.7	↓
HCO_3^- (mmol/L)	24.2	No change
Lactate (mmol/L)	5.9	↑↑↑

Table 4.6 Severe metabolic acidosis in severe pneumonia with sepsis

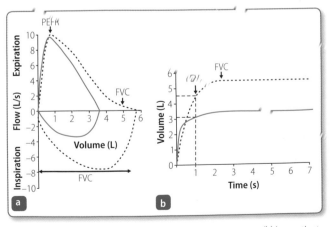

Figure 4.9 Typical flow-volume loop (a) and volume-time curve (b) in a patient with pneumonia (blue line). Dashed line = normal. FVC, forced vital capacity; PEFR, peak expiratory flow rate; FEV$_1$, forced expiratory volume in 1 second.

tachypnoea and characteristic end-inspiratory crackles heard on auscultation.

Chest radiography shows reduced volume of lungs and reticular micronodular and interstitial fibrosis. Computed tomography (CT) scanning may show thickened intra-alveolar septa, ground-glass haziness, and nodular and fibrotic patterns (**Figure 4.10**). Fibrosis of the alveolar–capillary membrane impairs gas exchange and the alveolar–arterial oxygen gradient ($P_{A-a}O_2$). Recent studies into interstitial diseases, however, have suggested that blood gas disturbances and symptoms are due more to loss of respiratory surface area and loss of capillary bed than to the diffusion impairment itself. However, monitoring the T_LCO has proven useful for diagnosis and assessing disease state.

Changes in lung function include:

- restrictive ventilatory impairment due to gradual loss of lung volume
- preservation of flow rates
- reduction in the T_LCO
- reduced compliance due to stiff non-distensible lungs with increased elastic recoil
- increased $P_{A-a}O_2$ gradient both at rest and on exercise
- dyspnoea caused by increased work of breathing and characterised by resting tachypnoea and small tidal volumes
- hypoxaemia and respiratory alkalosis which may be seen on ABG measurements

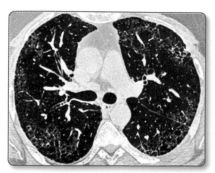

Figure 4.10 High-resolution CT scan of advanced stage of pulmonary fibrosis demonstrating reticular opacities with honeycombing, and predominant subpleural distribution.

In a typical person with exertional dyspnoea, the O_2 saturation at rest is normal, but marked O_2 desaturation occurs on exercise with a normal or low P_aCO_2. The ventilation tests are characterised

Clinical insight

Administration of O_2 at a tension slightly higher than normal may correct hypoxaemia and relieve dyspnoea completely.

by an often striking loss of VC and TLC. The RV may be reduced but usually not to the same degree as the other measured lung volumes. This frequently results in an elevated RV/TLC ratio. However, the normal FEV_1 as % FVC prevents confusion with obstructive emphysema.

Pulmonary compliance is invariably reduced to less than half normal. This means that there is an increase in the work of breathing against elastic resistance. The principal abnormality is a reduction in the diffusing capacity. Reduced lung volumes, hyperventilation and the absence of obstructive ventilatory disease, although important, are distinguishing features that are merely suggestive of disease.

4.3 Pulmonary vascular disease

Pulmonary vascular diseases involve the blood circulation within the lungs. They can be acute (as in the case of a pulmonary embolism) or more chronic as seen in pulmonary hypertension.

In most cases of pulmonary vascular disease there is a reduction in the T_LCO but often with normal lung volume, capacity and spirometry. However, in pulmonary haemorrhage, the T_LCO is increased due to blood within the alveolar space binding CO more strongly.

An elevated alveolar dead space/tidal volume (V_D/V_T) of > 45% in the absence of obstructive or restrictive disease suggests a vascular disease of the lungs.

Pulmonary embolism

A pulmonary embolus is a blood clot in the blood circulation of the lungs. This is a medical emergency and is categorised into three types:

- massive pulmonary embolism
- recurrent small pulmonary emboli
- pulmonary embolism with subsequent infarction

Sixty per cent of pulmonary circulation must be obliterated to produce signs of distress and 80% to cause death (**Figure 4.11**).

Pulmonary embolism is common in patients undergoing surgery who have restricted activity, infection and pulmonary congestion (often secondary to left-sided heart failure). Pulmonary thrombosis is likely to occur around small emboli when the flow is reduced, the vessel wall damaged and the state of blood renders clot formation easy.

ABGs in pulmonary embolism

ABGs can be helpful in making the diagnosis, although definitive investigation requires radiology such as a CT, pulmonary angiogram or ventilation–perfusion scan to visualise the clot. ABGs in the acute stage (**Table 4.7**) reflect an acute hypoxia and often show type I respiratory failure.

Occlusion of a part of the pulmonary circulation means that there are areas of alveoli that are not receiving blood,

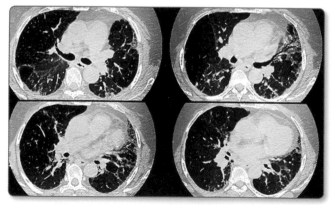

Figure 4.11 High-resolution segmental CT scans showing increased pulmonary attenuation with distortion of the pulmonary architecture in 4 segmental scans.

ABG measure	Level	Change
pH	7.39	No change
PCO_2 (kPa)	3.2	↓
PO_2 (kPa)	6.7	↓↓
HCO_3^- (mmol/L)	23.2	No change
Lactate (mmol/L)	0.7	No change

Table 4.7 Arterial blood gases in a significant pulmonary embolism.

i.e. alveolar dead space. A simple measure of dead space is to calculate the difference between P_aCO_2 and end-tidal P_aCO_2, which can be large in a severe embolisation. A fall in O_2 uptake in the affected lung and a decrease in the diffusing capacity occur. There is also a fall in lung compliance, although lung function testing is not usually carried out in the acute stages.

Primary pulmonary hypertension

Recurrent pulmonary embolism may occur in chronic illness, particularly in bed-ridden patients with heart disease. Multiple small pulmonary emboli can cause progressive primary pulmonary hypertension. Other causes of primary pulmonary hypertension are pulmonary schistosomiasis, polyarteritis nodosa and cancer.

Pulmonary haemorrhage

Pulmonary haemorrhage is often diagnosed on the basis of a clinical presentation of haemoptysis and florid changes on a chest radiograph or CT scan. Lung function tests are not advised because they may worsen the clinical situation. However, serial measurements of the T_LCO are safe to make and can be used to monitor clinical progress. A raised T_LCO with low haemoglobin in a patient with a characteristic clinical picture is sufficient to make the diagnosis.

4.4 Pleural disease

Pneumothorax

A pneumothorax is a collapsed lung. The diagnosis is made from a history of sudden pleuritic chest pain, decreased or absent breath sounds over the affected area, and a chest radiograph showing a pneumothorax (**Figure 4.12**).

Lung function testing is not carried out at any stage of acute primary disease. However, if the pneumothorax is secondary to an underlying lung condition, e.g. COPD, simple spirometry may be used to help diagnosis and to plan management. ABGs in a pneumothorax may reveal a degree of hypoxia with no other changes.

Pleural effusion

Pleural effusion is an increase in fluid within the lung's pleural space (**Figure 4.13**). Spirometry is carried out only if surgical management is to be contemplated as it gives a good indication of suitability for a major operation. ABGs in a major pleural effusion may show respiratory compromise with type I or type II respiratory failure.

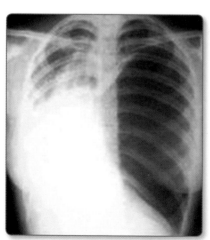

Figure 4.12 Chest radiograph showing a large spontaneous tension pneumothorax of the left side. Note the marked depression of the right hemidiaphragm and the mediastinal shift to the right, suggesting tension pneumothorax.

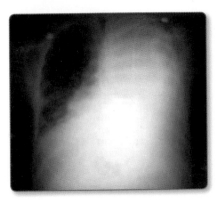

Figure 4.13
Posteroanterior upright chest radiograph showing a massive left-sided pleural effusion with contralateral mediastinal shift.

4.5 Chest wall disorders

Chest wall disorders are abnormalities in the physical structure of the chest wall. A chest deformity can limit thoracic size and expansion, thereby presenting a restrictive pattern on lung function tests. Test abnormalities include a low VC and lung volume, and full spirometry may reveal a restrictive defect with normal T_LCO. Common chest wall disorders producing a restrictive pattern are:

- kyphoscoliosis
- pectus carinum/excavatum
- surgery, e.g. thoracoplasty, plombage
- trauma, e.g. flail chest

Circulatory dysfunction

A number of cardiac diseases produce abnormalities in both lung function and ABG tests. Disorders that cause a decrease in functional blood flow (i.e. a decrease in the amount of blood available for tissues), such as anaemia, may result in a low PO_2. Conversely, disorders such as polycythaemia may show an overabundance of functional blood (in terms of a raised haemoglobin) which may result in a raised PO_2.

Other cardiac conditions such as cor pulmonale are a direct consequence of respiratory disease and lung function testing may reflect the underlying condition, e.g. the obstructive spirometry pattern of chronic obstructive pulmonary disease (COPD).

5.1 Changes in lung volume

VC is frequently decreased when there is pulmonary vascular congestion. RV may decrease together with the total lung capacity (TLC) in severe pulmonary congestion, but it is usually normal. The RV may be increased absolutely, not just relative to other volume compartments, when airway obstruction occurs from mucosal oedema or bronchial narrowing. This is a feature of acute left ventricular failure (cardiac asthma) or sudden pulmonary vascular obstruction (i.e. pulmonary embolism).

5.2 Changes in ventilation

Changes in alveolar ventilation are common in patients with heart disease. There is often hyperventilation, particularly with exercise. The excess ventilation is out of proportion to the oxygen need and causes a lowered P_aCO_2, with a rise in pH resulting in a compensated respiratory alkalosis. This disturbance of acid–base equilibrium is seen frequently in patients with chronic pulmonary vascular congestion and in some patients with congenital cyanotic heart disease.

Some patients with long-standing right-to-left shunts, who often have severe hypoxaemia, do not hyperventilate. Their ventilation may be lower than that of normal individuals living at high altitudes who have comparable degrees of hypoxia, i.e. those with long-standing shunts are better able to tolerate their hypoxia.

Some patients with terminal left ventricular failure are unable to hyperventilate despite severe hypoxaemia. This may occur when there is a marked decrease in compliance and obstruction to airflow due to severe pulmonary vascular congestion, oedema, swollen bronchial mucosa or broncho-spasm. These patients can sometimes develop CO_2 retention and respiratory acidosis due to hypoventilation. If the CO_2 retention becomes chronic the kidneys compensate by retaining bicarbonate.

5.3 Changes in perfusion

If the quantity of blood flow through anatomical shunts is increased, as occurs in congenital heart diseases with right-to-left shunt, the systemic arterial blood will be altered so that the O_2 content decreases and the CO_2 content increases.

With pulmonary oedema there may be severe alterations in the ratio of ventilation to perfusion ($\dot{V}/\dot{Q}$) and depending on the extent of oedema there will be regions of diminished flow with normal ventilation, areas of diminished ventilation with relatively normal flow, or both.

5.4 Changes in diffusion

The diffusing capacity might be expected to increase in diseases in which there is an excessive pulmonary capillary volume, because there is more haemoglobin available for gas transport. Indeed, this is often the case in the presence of left-to-right shunts, e.g. an atrial septal defect.

However, in other diseases in which there is increased pulmonary capillary volume, diffusing capacity decreases. This is true in mitral stenosis, where it may be due in part to thickening of the alveolar septa as the disease progresses: the diffusing capacity impairment parallels the severity of the mitral stenosis.

Diffusion may be increased in left ventricular failure because of the increased quantities of blood in the lungs. The reason is obscure but the lowered values may be due to decreased diffusion across oedematous alveolar septa or as a function of poor distribution of inspired gas within the alveoli in relation to blood flow.

In diseases of the pulmonary capillary bed and small pulmonary vessels, the diffusing capacity is generally normal. As the diseases progress with vessel wall thickening, elevated pulmonary vascular resistance and decreased pulmonary blood volume, the diffusion may fall. This also occurs in the late stages of right-to-left shunts with pulmonary hypertension.

> ### Guiding principle
>
> Gas transfer is dependent on haemoglobin availability, so conditions that affect haemoglobin levels will affect the T_LCO.

5.5 Cardiac diseases

Diseases of cardiac output

Acute left ventricular heart disease leading to pulmonary oedema may show an increase in RV due to airway obstruction. This arises due to both decreased lung compliance and obstruction by fluid. In more chronic left-sided heart disease the T_LCO may be increased due to the increased amount of blood in the lungs as a consequence of poor cardiac output.

Cor pulmonale is right-sided heart disease, secondary to increased resistance in the pulmonary circulation. The lung function abnormalities are those of the underlying disease. A patient with COPD as the underlying cause of cor pulmonale, for example, would probably have an obstructive

> ### Guiding principle
>
> Lung function investigations are not usually helpful in assessing patients with acute cardiac disease, but ABG testing may reveal a low PO_2 in patients who are unable to maintain adequate blood oxygenation due to their cardiac disease.

pattern on lung function tests (see **Figures 3.4** and **4.5**).

The diseases most likely to cause cor pulmonale are:
- COPD
- obstructive sleep apnoea
- sarcoidosis
- bronchopulmonary dysplasia
- sickle cell disease
- pulmonary embolism (causing an acute cor pulmonale)

ABGs in all forms of heart disease may show evidence of hypoxaemia with a low

Clinical insight

- The Framingham risk score is based on a long-term US study that started in 1948 and devised a number of cardiac markers to determine the risk of heart disease, e.g. systolic blood pressure and high-density lipoprotein (HDL)-cholesterol
- A number of studies have shown that a low FVC in patients at risk of heart disease is a useful marker of an increased risk
- The combination of FVC with the Framingham risk score is thought to provide an even more robust measure of risk of cardiac disease

PO_2. In the end-stages the resulting circulatory failure will cause an increasing PCO_2 and type II respiratory failure, as seen in **Table 5.1**.

Anaemia and shock

Anaemia or significant blood loss, as seen in shock, will decrease the T_LCO (in contrast to pulmonary haemorrhage which will cause an increase) because carbon monoxide transfer depends on haemoglobin levels in the blood. Anaemia generally presents with no changes on ABG results (**Table 5.2**). This is because,

ABG measure	Level	Change
pH	7.21	↓↓
PCO_2 (kPa)	11.2	↑
PO_2 (kPa)	4.6	↓↓
HCO_3^- (mmol/L)	23.4	No change
Sodium (mmol/L)	129	↓
Potassium (mmol/L)	5.8	↑

Table 5.1 Arterial blood gases in end-stage circulatory failure.

ABG measure	Level	Change
pH	7.43	No change
PCO_2 (kPa)	4.5	No change
PO_2 (kPa)	10.2	No change
HCO_3^- (mmol/L)	23.2	No change
Sodium (mmol/L)	139	No change
Potassium (mmol/L)	3.7	No change

Table 5.2 Arterial blood gases in anaemia.

although the reduction in haemoglobin reduces total oxygen content, the PO_2 is unchanged.

Carbon monoxide poisoning

Carbon monoxide (CO) combines with haemoglobin with a much higher affinity than O_2 (> 200-fold) and causes a left shift of the oxyhaemoglobin dissociation curve. An ABG analysis may show a normal PO_2 (as the PO_2 in the blood is independent of the amount bound to haemoglobin). Carboxyhaemoglobin levels may also be measured directly and shown to be elevated. Pulse oximetry may show incorrect PO_2 levels because simple oximeters incorrectly measure carboxyhaemoglobin as oxyhaemoglobin and hence a specific carboxyhaemoglobin monitoring device should be used. An example of ABGs in carbon monoxide poisoning is shown in **Table 5.3**.

ABG measure	Level	Change
pH	7.37	No change
PCO_2 (kPa)	4.2	No change
PO_2 (kPa)	10.7	No change
HCO_3^- (mmol/L)	22.9	No change

Table 5.3 Arterial blood gases in in carbon monoxide poisoning.

Polycythaemia

Polycythaemia is an abnormally high red blood cell content and has two forms: primary and secondary.

Primary polycythaemia (polycythaemia rubra vera) is due to an excess production of red blood cells as a consequence of a primary abnormality of the bone marrow. The elevated haemoglobin may lead to an increased $T_L CO$ on lung function testing due to the increased availability of haemoglobin to carry the gas, whereas the $P_a O_2$ may be normal.

Secondary polycythaemia is due to an increase in erythropoietin as a consequence of chronically low O_2 levels in the blood. Lung function tests and ABGs may reflect the underlying disease, e.g. an obstructive pattern seen in COPD. Causes of secondary polycythaemia include:

- iatrogenic, e.g. blood loss
- physiological, e.g. living at high altitude
- respiratory, e.g. COPD

Table 5.4 shows ABGs in a patient with polycythaemia secondary to COPD.

Congenital heart disease

Congenital heart diseases encompass a spectrum of diseases from minor conditions to those that are fatal shortly after birth. Assessments of children prior to corrective surgery may involve the use of ABG and lung function testing to investigate the severity of disease.

In patients born with a right-to-left shunt the systemic arterial blood reflects the mixing of arterial and venous blood

ABG measure	Level	Change
pH	7.42	No change
PCO_2 (kPa)	6.7	↑
PO_2 (kPa)	9.2	↓
HCO_3^- (mmol/L)	23.7	No change

Table 5.4 Arterial blood gases in polycythaemia secondary to copd.

ABG measure	Level	Change
pH	7.36	No change
PCO_2 (kPa)	6.5	↑
PO_2 (kPa)	8.2	↓
HCO_3^- (mmol/L)	23.2	No change

Table 5.5 Arterial blood gases in right-to-left shunting of blood.

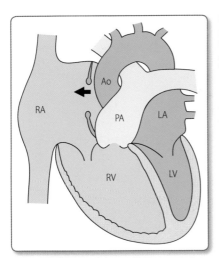

Figure 5.1 Inappropriate mixing of blood in a large atrial septal defect secundum (arrow). The right atrium (RA), right ventricle (RV) and pulmonary artery (PA) are enlarged. Ao, aorta; LA, left atrium; LV, left ventricle.

and may show a decreased PO_2 and increased PCO_2 (**Table 5.5**). In other congenital heart diseases there may be a low P_aCO_2 with a rise in pH.

Figure 5.1 shows the effect of communicating atrial compartments in a patient with an atrial septal defect. The increased pulmonary blood flow (from a left-to-right shunt) causes an increased T_LCO on lung function testing as a higher concentration of haemoglobin is passing through the pulmonary circulation.

Neuromuscular disorders

Respiratory disturbances in neuromuscular conditions can be due to abnormalities in
- the central nervous system
- muscle innervation or
- respiratory muscles

Some patients with these disorders may present with acute respiratory failure and abnormal ABGs, for example in the case of an acute haemorrhagic stroke. Other neuromuscular disorders may present with an acute exacerbation of a chronic disorder, or with chronic respiratory failure.

Lung function assessments in an acute-on-chronic neuromuscular condition can determine the respiratory reserve and hence assess the need for assisted ventilation. This also applies to ABGs showing either a type I or a type II respiratory failure.

Basic spirometry may show a restrictive lung pattern, with the severity of the disease displayed by the extent of the restriction. A number of additional lung function tests can be used to determine the type and severity of a neuromuscular disease, including:
- tilt-table testing, which can identify a diaphragm weakness
- mouth pressure measurements to isolate a myopathy
- sleep studies to confirm an obstructive sleep apnoea/hypopnoea syndrome (see Chapter 2).

6.1 Respiratory tests in management of neuromuscular disorders

Standard tests for pulmonary function can be used in the basic assessment of neurological disease affecting the lungs; however, neuromuscular weakness may impair a patient's ability to adequately perform lung function tests. Additional specialised tests are used when monitoring patients with significant neuromuscular weakness.

In practice, most hospitals use bedside hand-held spirometers to keep a record of the forced vital capacity (FVC) and ABGs to monitor patients admitted acutely with decompensated respiratory failure. Mouth pressure and sleep study tests are also useful in monitoring the progress of respiratory function in neuromuscular diseases, usually in an outpatient setting.

Lung function tests are also useful in patients with neuromuscular disease, in the monitoring of respiratory fitness and, over a period of time, progression of the disease. Thus, they may prove useful in management.

Spirometry

Spirometry, in addition to blood gases, is invaluable in respiratory failure due to an underlying neurological problem. Small hand-held devices are preferable because they can be easily used on the ward, allowing instant recording of FVC. Slow vital capacity (SVC) can be measured if physical weakness or coughing makes assessment of FVC inappropriate.

The usual patterns seen in patients with neuromuscular diseases are restrictive: reduced forced expiratory volume in 1 second (FEV_1) as well as a reduced FVC (FEV_1/FVC ratio is > 70%) (see **Figure 3.5**). Occasionally it may be possible to detect mixed obstructive as well as restrictive disorders (FEV_1/FVC ratio is < 70% and the FVC is < 80% predicted). Monitoring lung function is useful in assessment of disease state as well as in setting therapeutic targets.

> **Clinical insight**
>
> - Patients with an acute or acute-on-chronic exacerbation of neurological disease may need urgent intubation and ventilation
> - A sudden drop in the FVC or deteriorating ABG measurements (e.g. indicating type II respiratory failure) are all indications for ventilatory support

Arterial blood gases

The frequency of ABG monitoring required in neuromuscular disease depends on the severity of respiratory compromise resulting from loss of respiratory muscle function.

Mouth pressures

Mouth pressure readings can be helpful in assessing the level of neuromuscular disease; methods of measuring them are described in Chapter 2. The VC supine is normally within 5% of the VC erect and a drop of over 25% is considered abnormal. In respiratory muscle weakness, a patient may display a low TLC and FVC with an increased RV and $T_L$co.

The maximum inspiratory pressure (MIP) and maximum expiratory pressure (MEP) readings are useful in neuromuscular disorders because the deviation from normal values corresponds with disease severity. MIP and MEP values seen in various conditions are given in **Table 6.1**.

Sleep studies

Sleep studies are indicated for the assessment of patients with neuromuscular disorders such as central sleep apnoea. The method of testing and the interpretation of results are discussed in detail in Chapters 2 and 4.

	Maximal inspiratory pressure	Maximal expiratory pressure
Poor effort	Decreased	Decreased
Myopathy (myasthenia)	Decreased	Decreased
Neurological	Decreased	Decreased
Large volumes (obstructive lung diseases)	Decreased	Normal
Small volumes (restrictive lung diseases)	Normal	Decreased

Table 6.1 Changes in mouth pressure in different circumstances.

Commonly in neuromuscular weakness, hypopnoea (shallow breathing with a low respiratory rate) occurs. However, if the patient develops brain-stem disease (e.g. in motor neuron disease), there are central apnoeic episodes, obstructive episodes and hypopnoea due to bulbar muscle weakness.

Tilt testing

Tilt testing is indicated in patients who have neuromuscular disorders, for example diaphragm weakness. The methods of testing are described in detail in Chapter 2. Patterns of change in tilt-table results are shown in **Table 6.2**.

A significant drop in VC, with ensuing fall in O_2 saturation and paradoxical respiration (i.e. the abdomen moves in with inspiration rather than moving out), is strongly suggestive of diaphragm weakness (**Table 6.2**). In orthodeoxia there is a

	Vital capacity	Paradoxical respiration	Desaturation	Respiratory rate
Diaphragm weakness	Lowered on supine position	Yes, when supine	Yes, on supine position	Increases when supine
Intra-abdominal disease	Lowered on supine position	None seen	Yes, on supine position	Increases slightly when supine
Orthodeoxia/platypnoea	Normal in both erect and supine positions	None seen	Improves on laying supine	Decreases when supine
Orthopnoea due to heart failure/airway obstruction	Normal or increased in both erect and supine positions	None seen	Yes, on supine position	Increases when supine

Table 6.2 Changes during tilt-table testing.

normal VC and respiratory movement, and desaturation occurs on the upright position and improves on lying flat.

Platypnoea orthodeoxia is a rare syndrome of postural hypoxaemia accompanied by breathlessness. The predominant symptom, dyspnoea, induced by upright posture, can be debilitating and difficult to discern without thorough evaluation of the pattern of dyspnoea. The precise cause of the syndrome is unclear but patients develop right-to-left intracardiac shunting in the presence of normal right-sided cardiac pressures.

6.2 Motor neuron disease

Motor neuron disease (MND) is one of a spectrum of disorders in which progressive neurological damage results in problems with basic muscle activity such as that required for walking, moving, breathing and swallowing. The symptoms are due to disruptions in the neuronal signal pathways from the brain stem and spinal cord to the muscles. Common forms of MND include:

- amyotrophic lateral sclerosis (ALS)
- primary lateral sclerosis
- progressive muscular atrophy
- progressive bulbar palsy

MNDs can be inherited or acquired and symptoms in adults often appear after the age of 40 years. The inherited forms of MND can present in the first few years of life.

The disease is ultimately fatal as bulbar symptoms and signs progress. Death is usually due to respiratory failure, aspiration pneumonia and complications of prolonged immobility.

Lung function tests in MND

Lung function testing in all stages of disease reveals a restrictive defect and decline in FVC (see **Figure 3.5**), with corresponding type II respiratory failure seen on ABGs (**Table 6.3**). Overnight oximetry/sleep studies can reveal nocturnal hypoxia, which may require oxygen and palliative nasal ventilator support.

ABG measure	Level	Change
pH	7.24	↓↓
PCO_2 (kPa)	8.8	↑↑
PO_2 (kPa)	6.2	↓↓
HCO_3^- (mmol/L)	24.1	No change

Table 6.3 Arterial blood gas changes in acute-on-chronic motor neuron disease.

Serial measurements are taken over time to indicate improvement or decline after therapeutic interventions. The most common measurement used in the hospital setting is the FVC. In acute presentations FVC is measured regularly (e.g. every 2 hours). A drop in FVC by 50% predicted or the patient's best on admission indicates that the patient may need intubation.

6.3 Myasthenia gravis

Myasthenia gravis is an autoimmune disorder in which auto-antibodies to the acetylcholine receptor of the neuromuscular junction cause fluctuating muscle weakness. The pathognomonic feature of disease is muscle weakness that increases during activity and improves after periods of rest. Muscle groups that are commonly involved include those of facial expression such as the eyes and eyelids, as well as those of talking and swallowing. Muscles controlling ventilation may also be involved.

Lung function tests in myasthenia gravis

In myasthenia gravis the FVC is often low, so it is important to know the individual's baseline FVC (**Table 6.4**) to see how severe the lung defect is. Forced expirograph tests show a pattern similar to that of a restrictive lung defect (see **Figure 3.5**). Spirometry is carried out if the patient presents in respiratory failure during a myasthenic crisis and also when steroids are first administered as they can cause an initial worsening of

Month	January	February	March	April
FEV$_1$ (L)	1.7	1.6	2.1	1.9
FVC (L)	2.3	2.1	2.4	2.2
FEV$_1$, forced expiratory volume in 1 second; FVC, forced vital capacity.				

Table 6.4 Monthly lung function change in fluctuating myasthenia gravis.

symptoms for 1–2 weeks. Daily spirometry can therefore be a good guide to the state of clinical stability. It is not uncommon for a patient with myasthenia to be given drugs that increase the risk of respiratory failure, e.g. aminoglycosides, which increase the neuromuscular blockade.

Lambert–Eaton myasthenic syndrome (LEMS) is rare variant of the disease. It presents with features similar to myasthenia gravis, except that respiratory involvement is unusual and the disease is worse in the morning and improves with exercise. About 50% of cases have underlying small cell carcinoma of the lung. ABGs in some cases may indicate a type II respiratory failure, similar to that seen in **Table 6.3.**

6.4 Guillain–Barré syndrome

Guillain–Barré syndrome is an acute inflammatory demyelinating polyneuropathy that affects the peripheral nervous system. It often occurs shortly after a respiratory or gastrointestinal viral infection, which acts as the trigger. Initial symptoms may include distal weakness and tingling, which may spread to the central body. In severe cases this may lead to a total paralysis, with the loss of respiratory muscles causing respiratory arrest.

Reflexes, including knee jerks, are usually lost and a nerve conduction test showing a slowed velocity due to demyelination may give clues to the diagnosis. There may also be an increased protein level in the cerebrospinal fluid (CSF).

The Miller–Fisher variant presents with cranial nerve palsies and respiratory failure is an increased risk. These patients initially require FVC monitoring every 2 hours and a fall of 50%

predicted (or baseline if known) is considered an indication to intubate. An FVC of 15 mL/kg also indicates intubation. ABGs in severe disease may show a type II respiratory failure, similar to that seen in **Table 6.3**.

6.5 Diaphragm palsy

Diaphragm paralyses encompass a spectrum of disorders including either unilateral or bilateral diaphragmatic paralyses (**Table 6.5**). Many causes of unilateral paralyses may be found incidentally because they cause no noticeable respiratory symptoms other than dyspnoea on exertion. Examination may reveal dullness to percussion and absent breath sounds over the lower chest on the involved side.

In bilateral paralysis, patients are symptomatic and the disorder may reflect a more severe underlying lung pathology. The accessory respiratory muscles take over some of the function of the diaphragm. However, the increased work of these muscles may not be enough to maintain adequate respiration, leading to ventilatory failure and ultimately respiratory arrest. ABGs in severe disease may show a type II respiratory failure similar to that seen in **Table 6.3**.

Other symptoms include insomnia, morning headaches and excessive daytime sleepiness. Chest examination

Clinical scenario

A 37-year-old woman with no significant medical past is admitted to the emergency ward after a 4-day history of progressive weakness in her legs, moving towards her abdomen and her chest. She complains of 3 hours of increasing difficulty with breathing and her family reports a mild acute confusion. Her lung function testing shows a reduced FVC.

The story fits with Guillain–Barré syndrome but the differential should include Miller–Fisher variant, viral meningitis, Lyme disease, botulism, cytomegalovirus (CMV), MND, myasthenia gravis and space-occupying lesion.

The immediate investigations include:
- a full infection screen
- ABGs
- brain imaging
- lumbar puncture for CSF analysis
- nerve conduction studies
- spirometry

If the diagnosis of Guillain–Barré syndrome is suspected, the criteria for immediate critical care assessment with subsequent intubation and ventilation include an FVC of < 50% predicted or type II respiratory failure.

Site of lesion	Differential diagnosis
Spinal cord	Transection above C5 Multiple sclerosis Severe spondylosis
Motor neuron	Amyotrophic lateral sclerosis Spinal muscular atrophy Polymyositis Poliomyelitis
Phrenic nerve	Neuralgic amyotrophy Guillain–Barré polyneuropathy Charcot–Marie–Tooth disease Trauma (blunt/cold injury) Malignant invasion Paraneoplastic lesion
Diaphragmatic muscle	Acid maltase deficiency Myasthenia gravis Limb–girdle dystrophy Systemic lupus erythematosus Mixed connective tissue disease Systemic sclerosis Amyloidosis Hypothyroidism

Table 6.5 Aetiology of diaphragm palsy.

reveals a limitation of diaphragmatic excursions and bilateral lower chest dullness with absent breath sounds; on close inspection there will be a paradoxical inward movement of the abdomen on inspiration.

Lung function tests in diaphragm palsy

Patients who go on to develop severe restrictive ventilatory impairment may have a VC and TLC < 50% predicted. Lung capacity is reduced further when the patient assumes the supine position,

Guiding principle

Ventilation is initiated by negative intrathoracic pressure due in part to movement of the diaphragm, resulting in expansion of the ribcage and movement of gases from the atmosphere into the lungs. Innervation of the diaphragm is via the phrenic nerves, which leave the spinal cord at the level of C3–C5.

which explains why some patients become more dyspnoeic when lying down or even when swimming.

Spirometry reveals a restrictive defect that falls by 20% or more on lying flat. Overnight oximetry/sleep studies are required to see if nasal ventilation is needed. Further tests include:

- sniff/twitch testing, in which a positive result is a paradoxical elevation of a paralysed diaphragm in inspiration, as seen on fluoroscopy
- diaphragm stimulation, in which the phrenic nerve is electrically stimulated to see if it is still intact

6.6 Myopathies

Myopathies are neuromuscular disorders characterised by muscle weakness, which results from muscle fibre dysfunction.

One example is myotonic dystrophy, which is the most common cause of muscular dystrophy in adults. It presents as a slowly progressive multisystem disease affecting a wide range of muscles, including cardiac, gastrointestinal, smooth muscle and respiratory muscles.

A number of myopathies manifest in early childhood, e.g. Duchenne muscular dystrophy. Becker muscular dystrophy cases can also present in late childhood.

FVC monitoring (**Table 6.6**) and sleep studies may be useful to guide interventions in myopathic patients.

6.7 Vocal cord paralysis

Vocal cord paralysis can occur due to a number of acute factors such as viral infection, chemical irritants or extreme stress, or

Month	January	February	March	April
FEV_1 (L)	1.7	1.6	1.4	1.2
FVC (L)	2.3	2.1	1.7	1.5
FEV_1, forced expiratory volume in 1 s; FVC, forced vital capacity.

Table 6.6 Monthly lung function change in worsening muscular dystrophy.

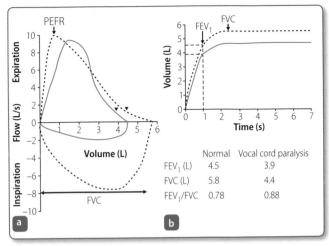

Figure 6.1 Flow-volume loops (a) and forced expirographs (b) with traces representing predicted (dashed) and vocal cord paralysis (blue) results. PEFR, peak expiratory flow rate; FEV_1, forced expiratory volume in 1 second (arrowheads); FVC, forced vital capacity.

during more chronic conditions such as upper airway cancer. Diagnosis is often made by direct visualisation of the vocal cords using a laryngoscope.

One of the differential diagnoses is asthma, so flow–volume loops can be used to distinguish between the two disorders. In vocal cord paralysis, the FVC often decreases together with the FEV_1 (a finding that is not seen during an asthma exacerbation) and flow–volume loops show flattening of the inspiratory loop (**Figure 6.1**).

6.8 Trauma and chest wall deformities

Trauma to the chest can cause a number of abnormalities in lung function. Typically mild trauma may result in a reduction in peak flow, FEV and FVC as observed by spirometry. More serious trauma can result in a flail chest, where a segment of the chest wall becomes detached from the rest of the chest and begins to move independently. A flail chest is a life-threatening surgical emergency requiring chest tube drainage, analgesia and ventilation.

In all cases of chest wall trauma there may be a reduction in O_2 saturation as well as a derangement of blood gases. The level of hypoxia is related to the level of trauma and it may initially show a type I respiratory failure, but progress to a type II respiratory failure in more severe disease (**Table 6.7**).

Spinal deformity can constrict lung as well as thoracic cavity size and inspiration ability. Spirometry shows a restrictive defect and some patients with severe disease require long-term O_2 therapy.

6.9 Neuroactive drugs

A number of drugs that act as respiratory stimulants or depressants are listed in **Table 6.8**. In some of these the effect is intended, whereas in others, e.g. salicylates, it is an unwanted side effect. Others (e.g. doxapram) are used specifically to stimulate the respiratory system before or as an adjunct to assisted ventilation. They can cause a variety of abnormalities in both lung function and blood gases, but in general most stimulants cause a level of immediate hyperventilation that results in a low P_aCO_2 and an elevated P_aO_2. If this continues the patient may fatigue, leading to hypoxaemia and hypercapnia.

ABG measure	Level	Change
pH	7.32	↓
PCO_2 (kPa)	9.3	↑↑
PO_2 (kPa)	4.2	↓↓
HCO_3^- (mmol/L)	22.1	No change

Table 6.7 Arterial blood gases in severe chest wall trauma.

Drugs that act as stimulants	Drugs that act as depressants
Acetazolamide	Alcohol
Aminophyllines	Anaesthetics
BIMU-8	Anticholinergics
Doxapram	Antihistamines
Prethcamide	Barbiturates
Progesterone	Benzodiazepines
Salicylates	Opiates

Table 6.8 Respiratory stimulants and depressants.

A number of drugs (e.g. benzodiazepines) have mild respiratory depressant effects as part of their primary use, but they can cause significant problems when taken in overdose. Other drugs (e.g. anaesthetics) are used primarily to induce anaesthesia for operations or to keep patients sedated while in intensive care, and they may subsequently depress the respiratory system.

> **Guiding principle**
>
> In general, respiratory depressants cause a level of central hypoventilation, which can lead to type I and then type II respiratory failure, with some patients needing intubation and ventilation.

6.10 Cerebrovascular accidents

The level of hypoxia seen in ABGs is usually related to the severity of the stroke. Patients who have an acute stroke may develop sudden-onset type I or II respiratory failure depending on which part of the brain has been affected by the stroke. However, in small strokes this hypoxia may be independent of the location of the infarct. This is due to the complex nature of the neurological control of breathing (see **Chapter 1**).

ABG measure	Level	Change
pH	7.34	↓
PCO_2 (kPa)	4.3	No change
PO_2 (kPa)	8.2	↓↓
HCO_3^- (mmol/L)	22.7	No change

Table 6.9 Arterial blood gases in acute stroke.

As with all acute neurological diseases requiring ventilatory support, the level of support given must be balanced against the patient's wishes and the long-term prognosis. An example of ABG levels in an acute stroke causing mild acidaemia and hypoxaemia is shown in **Table 6.9**.

Metabolic, endocrine and renal dysfunction

Diseases that affect the metabolic, endocrine and renal systems usually cause a metabolic acidosis with a subsequent respiratory attempt at compensation.

The arterial blood gases (ABGs) may indicate the intensity of disease. An ABG test showing a low pH and high lactate may indicate an acute and severe underlying disease. As such, ABGs are one of the key aspects of recognising a patient needing critical care.

In addition to the level of acidosis, ABGs are useful in providing a rapid measure of key electrolytes in some disorders. The blood potassium level may be dangerously high in acute renal failure or the initial stages of diabetic ketoacidosis, and serial repeated ABGs (taken to assess the metabolic and respiratory state) can help to assess this.

Lung function testing is not usually helpful in the acute management of metabolic, endocrine and renal disorders. However, it can help provide useful long-term information about co-morbidities and the level of

> ### Guiding principle
>
> ABG tests are useful in the acute phase of metabolic, endocrine and renal diseases to determine the level of metabolic shift and level of respiratory compensation, and assess the severity of an illness.

management needed. For example, a patient with end-stage chronic obstructive pulmonary disease (COPD) and poor lung function who presents with acute-on-chronic renal failure may not be suitable for long-term dialysis.

7.1 Diabetic ketoacidosis

Diabetic ketoacidosis (DKA) is a medical emergency that results from a shortage of insulin in patients with diabetes, leading to the metabolism of fatty acids and the production of ketones in the body (**Figure 7.1**). DKA may be the initial presentation in a subclinical diabetic and is often triggered by an unrelated factor such as an infection.

Despite the acute nature of DKA and its associated morbidity, an accurate assessment of the metabolic state and respiratory levels of compensation will facilitate successful intervention and rapid recovery of the patient. ABGs in the acute phase reflect a severe metabolic acidosis with some partial respiratory correction as the patient improves.

Although there are differences in the disease mechanisms, the results of some of the investigations seen in DKA are similar to those found in hyperosmotic non-ketotic (HONK) coma, which needs to remain in the differential diagnosis, particularly in older patients with established diabetes.

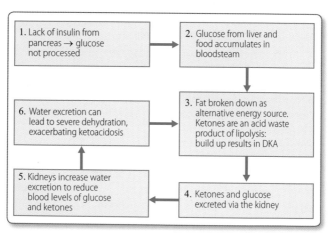

Figure 7.1 Ketone production in the body of a patient with diabetes. DKA, diabetic ketoacidosis.

Management of DKA should follow detailed local clinical guidelines and be done in conjunction with critical care teams where necessary.

Typical ABGs in diabetic ketoacidosis

Tables 7.1 and 7.2 show typical examples, the first in an acute situation and the second in a patient who is less severely ill.

Acute severe DKA

Table 7.1 shows ABGs in a patient with severe DKA metabolic acidosis. Severe acidosis is indicated by a very low pH together with a low bicarbonate. Clinically, the patient will often be hyperventilating, initially with rapid and shallow breaths but evolving to deep, laboured breathing (known as *Kussmaul's breathing*), in attempted respiratory compensation. The increased respiratory rate leads to a very high PO_2 and a very low PCO_2. However, there can be a delay in any reversal of the ketoacidosis as the system is overwhelmed by the levels of acidic ketone bodies.

In severe DKA, ABGs show a high glucose with electrolyte disturbances (hyperkalaemia, in this case). Hyperglycaemia is what differentiates DKA from other rarer forms of ketoacidosis, as the tissues are unable to utilise blood sugar. The hyperkalaemia

ABG measure	Level	Change
pH	7.14	↓↓↓
PCO_2 (kPa)	2.6	↓↓↓
PO_2 (kPa)	18.9	↑↑↑
HCO_3^- (mmol/L)	17.1	↓↓
Sodium (mmol/L)	133	↓
Potassium (mmol/L)	5.7	↑
Glucose (mmol/L)	36.2	↑↑↑

Table 7.1 Arterial blood gases in severe diabetic ketoacidosis.

ABG measure	Level	Change
pH	7.31	↓
PCO_2 (kPa)	4.4	↓
PO_2 (kPa)	14.4	↑
HCO_3^- (mmol/L)	18.1	↓
Sodium (mmol/L)	131	↓
Potassium (mmol/L)	4.6	No change
Glucose (mmol/L)	14.2	↑

Table 7.2 Arterial blood gases in a compensated diabetic ketoacidosis (with oxygen supplementation)

is the result of the excess extracellular hydrogen ions being exchanged for intracellular potassium. Hypokalaemia and hyponatraemia are also common, as electrolytes follow the excess glucose into the urine (osmotic diuresis).

Appropriate management results in the ABGs gradually reverting to normal over time. However, patients who do not respond well to treatment may become too unwell to maintain an increased respiratory rate, as may patients for whom appropriate care is delayed. Slowing of the respiratory rate results in a drop in PO_2 and rise in PCO_2, along with the existing acidosis. This situation of decompensation has a high mortality rate and critical care management should be initiated immediately. Patients who improve will slowly start to reverse their acidotic state with the

Clinical insight

- Patients with DKA are often severely dehydrated and fluids must be replaced swiftly but carefully in order to avoid cardiac decompensation, which is a greater risk in patients who may have diabetic macrovascular disease
- Fluid input and output should be accurately monitored
- Although the initial potassium levels may be high, insulin will drive potassium back into cells, leading to hypokalaemia and the associated risks of arrhythmias. ABGs provide accurate electrolyte measurements, but should not be taken solely for this purpose. Instead, phlebotomy is a less invasive method.

associated return to normal of the PO_2 and PCO_2.

Less acute DKA

Table 7.2 shows an example of partially compensated metabolic acidosis in a patient who is less unwell than the patient (see **Table 7.1**).

In less acute DKA, a common initial presentation is slightly low pH and low bicarbonate, indicating an acute metabolic acidosis. Respiratory compensation leads to high PO_2 and low PCO_2. Successful compensation results in a pH that is normal or only slightly low, along with high glucose levels. As less compensation is required, there is no hyperkalaemia, unlike more acute acidosis.

The very nature of a ketotic state means that patients in the acute phase of DKA may have a severe acidosis in which attempts at respiratory compensation are not initially successful. The pH may be lower than 7.0 in cases of medical emergency. In such instances, patients do not need supplementary O_2 if they have highly elevated PO_2 with a very low PCO_2.

Clinical scenario

A 19-year-old woman is admitted to the accident and emergency department in a drowsy state after a blood sugar reading by her general practitioner showing 'high'. Her ABG on room air shows:

- pH 7.12
- PCO_2 2.3 kPa
- PO_2 18.2 kPa
- bicarbonate 10.6 mmol/L
- blood glucose 38.3 mmol/L

The blood gas and clinical picture are consistent with a severe metabolic acidosis in a patient with newly diagnosed diabetes. The underlying cause of the acidosis is the production of ketones as a by-product of fatty acid metabolism. The initial goal is stabilisation with adequate fluid resuscitation and monitoring. Further immediate measures include reduction of her blood glucose levels with intravenous insulin and potassium supplementation when needed. Later goals of management include heparin prophylaxis, investigation and management of any initiating factor such as an underlying infection.

ABGs during management of diabetic ketoacidosis

The mainstay of DKA management is to reverse the metabolic state; this is primarily achieved with fluids to compensate for the severe dehydration on admission. Insulin is given as a bolus and then as a sliding scale to help bring down the glucose levels, and a number of other management plans are initiated, including thromboprophylaxis and treatment of any associated infection.

Patients who do not improve may become too unwell to maintain the increased respiratory rate. This will result in a slowing of the rate and a subsequent drop in PO_2 and rise in PCO_2, compounding the existing acidosis. This situation has a high mortality rate and critical care management should be initiated immediately. Patients who improve will slowly start to reverse their acidotic state with the associated return to normal of the PO_2 and PCO_2.

7.2 Conn's syndrome

Conn's syndrome is due to an oversecretion of aldosterone from the adrenal glands as a result of a solitary benign adrenal adenoma. The oversecretion leads to hypertension, muscle cramps and weakness.

ABGs can be helpful in making the diagnosis and show high sodium, low potassium and metabolic alkalosis, as seen in **Table 7.3**. These abnormalities arise from the action of aldosterone on the distal tubule of the kidney, which causes sodium reabsorption with a corresponding potassium and hydrogen ion secretion (**Figure 7.2**).

ABG measure	Level	Change
pH	7.52	↑↑
PCO_2 (kPa)	4.3	↓
PO_2 (kPa)	14.3	↑↑
HCO_3^- (mmol/L)	28.1	↑
Sodium (mmol/L)	129	↓
Potassium (mmol/L)	5.6	↑

Table 7.3 Arterial blood gases in Conn's syndrome.

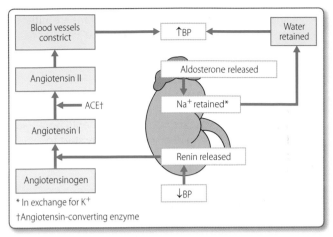

Figure 7.2 The renin–angiotensin–aldosterone system, which regulates blood pressure (BP), is affected by diuretic use.

7.3 Lactic acidosis

Lactic acidosis is an accumulation of lactic acid in tissues and blood, usually from excessive anaerobic respiration in skeletal muscles (**Table 7.4**).

Typical ABGs in lactic acidosis

Normal blood lactate concentration is 0.5–1.0 mmol/L and higher levels with associated acidosis reflect a higher severity of lactic acidosis. **Table 7.5** shows an example of a metabolic acidosis with raised lactate. The pH is low and the associated low bicarbonate indicates that there is a severe acute acidosis. The

> **Clinical insight**
>
> There are two forms of lactic acid: L-lactic acid is produced by humans and is what is measured in hospital laboratories; D-lactic acid is produced by bacteria, and high levels may reflect a metabolic acidosis due to bowel disease.

Direct hypoxia	Metabolic	Drugs	Genetic
Shock Tissue ischaemia Exercise Severe anaemia	Diabetic ketoacidosis Liver disease Neoplasms Renal failure	Alcohol Methanol poisoning Metformin Phenytoin Isoniazid Cocaine Biguanides	Glycogen storage disorders Pyruvate dehydrogenase deficiency Fructose-1,6-diphosphatase deficiency MELAS syndrome

MELAS, mitochondrial myopathy, encephalopathy, lactic acidosis and stroke.

Table 7.4 Causes of lactic acidosis.

ABG measure	Level	Change
pH	7.28	↓↓
PCO_2 (kPa)	2.4	↓↓
PO_2 (kPa)	13.7	↑
HCO_3^- (mmol/L)	16.8	↓
Lactate (mmol/L)	5.3	↑↑

Table 7.5 Arterial blood gases in lactic acidosis.

gas values show an attempt at compensation by an increase in respiratory rate.

7.4 Renal failure

Renal failure can usually be classified as acute (resulting in both elevated urea and creatinine levels) or chronic (with a high level of creatinine only). Patients with acute renal failure are metabolically more unstable than those with chronic renal failure who have been able to partially or fully physiologically compensate their metabolic state.

The causes of renal failure can be categorised according to whether the location of the pathology is before the kidney, within the kidney or after the kidney (**Table 7.6**). Broadly

Pre-renal	Renal	Post renal
Severe hypotension Sepsis Cardiac disease	Drugs, e.g. non-steroidal anti-inflammatory drugs Toxins, e.g. contrast reagent Acute tubular necrosis Acute interstitial nephritis Glomerulonephritis	Trauma Bladder tumour Kidney stones Prostate enlargement

Table 7.6 Causes of renal failure.

speaking *pre-renal failure* is due to a reduction in blood flow into the kidney, *renal failure* is due to kidney damage and *post-renal failure* is due to an outflow obstruction.

Metabolic acidosis in a patient with renal failure who is acutely ill

Table 7.7 shows an example of a severe metabolic acidosis in a patient who has renal failure and is acutely unwell. ABGs in this scenario reflect the level of sepsis and build-up of toxins, which the kidneys are unable to excrete. The pH is low and, together with the low bicarbonate,

Guiding principle

- A patient can have a relatively normal creatinine and still have lost a great deal of intrinsic renal function
- Investigations for further defining the type of renal failure include ultrasonography, eGFR (estimated glomerular filtration rate) and renal angiograms

ABG measure	Level	Change
pH	7.14	↓↓↓
PCO_2 (kPa)	3.2	↓
PO_2 (kPa)	13.1	↑
HCO_3^- (mmol/l)	17.3	↓
Sodium (mmol/L)	133	↓
Potassium (mmol/L)	5.9	↑↑

Table 7.7 Arterial blood gases in acute renal failure.

Clinical scenario

A 63-year-old man who was previously fit and well is assessed in A&E and given a diagnosis of left lower lobe pneumonia. He is found to be clinically dehydrated with deranged blood tests, including:

- raised white cell count (WCC)
- raised C-reactive protein (CRP)
- urea 23 mg/dL
- creatinine 93 µmol/L

His ABG on room air shows:

- pH 7.25
- PCO_2 2.7 kPa
- PO_2 16.2 kPa
- bicarbonate 14.6 mmol/L

The blood gas and clinical pictures are consistent with a severe metabolic acidosis. The trigger factor is the pneumonia; the raised urea with relatively normal creatinine points to an acute renal failure with sepsis from the pneumonia, making it pre-renal failure. The initial goal is to adequately rehydrate the patient and treat the underlying pneumonia with appropriate intravenous antibiotics. The blood gases and renal function should continue to be monitored and, if they deteriorate further or the patient has a poor urine output despite adequate rehydration, then a form of renal support such as emergency haemofiltration will be needed.

Guiding principle

The severity of metabolic acidosis, and the level of hyperkalaemia as determined by an ABG in acute renal failure, can be used to determine the need for emergency haemodialysis.

this indicates that there is a significant acidosis. The deranged gas values show that the patient is attempting to compensate for this acidosis by increasing the respiratory rate but this has yet to be successful. The remaining results show a slightly low sodium but a very high potassium. This level is probably acute and will need to be reduced urgently to prevent cardiac instability. Acute renal failure may result in severe metabolic acidosis which may require a form of temporary renal support such as emergency haemodialysis in a critical care unit.

Other disorders

A number of unique and unusual situations that have not been discussed in previous chapters can affect both the acid–base status and the lung function. As well as being of academic interest, they reflect real-life scenarios that are encountered on a daily basis in clinical practice, hence their inclusion here.

Although some disorders have characteristic arterial blood gas (ABG) or lung function disturbances (e.g. hyperventilating patients with anxiety disorders), others may be less easily identified, such as patterns of metabolic disturbances associated with vomiting.

8.1 Anxiety, pain and hyperventilation

In hyperventilation, increased ventilation results in blowing off CO_2 by the lungs, in turn resulting in respiratory alkalosis. Causes include:

- anxiety
- stress
- pain
- head injury or stroke
- extreme exercise
- aspirin overdose (which can also cause a metabolic acidosis)

Some patents presenting with anxiety and pain may show symptoms of hyperventilation, which can affect both lung function (by displaying an artificially low PEFR) and ABG status (which shows a respiratory alkalosis).

Hyperventilation is not diagnosed by ABG testing. Instead diagnosis is made from a supportive history and clinical context, with reliable measures of O_2 saturation using a pulse oximeter. However, if ABGs are measured in hyperventilation, they usually show hyperoxaemia, hypocapnia and a high pH.

Table 8.1 shows an example of ABGs in hyperventilation with a high PO_2 and a subsequent alkalosis. The bicarbonate is normal which reflects the acuteness of the respiratory alkalosis.

ABG measure	Level	Change
pH	7.52	↑
PCO_2 (kPa)	2.6	↓↓
PO_2 (kPa)	16.9	↑↑
HCO_3^- (mmol/L)	22.2	No change
Sodium (mmol/L)	137	No change
Potassium (mmol/L)	4.3	No change

Table 8.1 Arterial blood gases in hyperventilation.

Figure 8.1 shows the cycle of hyperventilation. An increased respiratory rate causes an increase in PO_2 and a decrease in PCO_2 which ultimately leads to exacerbation of the hyperventilation.

The treatment of hyperventilation involves first treating the cause, whether this is treatment for a head injury, behavioural exercises to relieve stress or appropriate pain management.

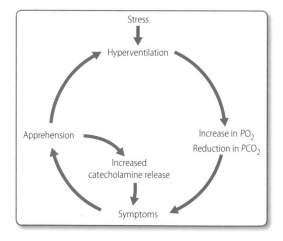

Figure 8.1 Hyperventilation cycle.

For patients with pure respiratory alkalosis, the management is to simply stop the hyperventilation. Breathing in and out of a paper bag may help increase the PCO_2 in the blood and thus reduce the level of ventilation. Some patients may require medication such as benzodiazepines to slow the rate of breathing to normal, but care must be taken to ensure that there

Clinical insight

Aspirin stimulates the brain stem respiratory centre and in the early stages of overdose can cause hyperventilation with a respiratory alkalosis. In larger doses aspirin can lead to the accumulation of pyruvic and lactic acids, causing a high gap metabolic acidosis.

Aspirin (salicylate) poisoning can therefore present with ABGs showing either a respiratory alkalosis or a metabolic acidosis.

is no overdose and to avoid dependency. Patients may also paradoxically need supplemental oxygen to calm them down and thus reduce the level of ventilation.

In the case of acute pain, the ABG profile of an acute respiratory alkalosis secondary to hyperventilation may be complicated by a coexisting metabolic acidosis linked to the cause of the pain, e.g. a lactic acidosis found after acute tissue trauma. The slow deep breaths that occur due to metabolic acidosis are called Kussmaul's breathing.

8.2 Vomiting and nasogastric suction

Patients with acute or chronic vomiting can present with either an acidosis or an alkalosis, the determination of which may help narrow down the differential diagnosis.

Patients who vomit continuously may develop a metabolic alkalosis (**Table 8.2**). The mechanism for this is the significant loss of hydrochloric acid from the stomach. The net bicarbonate gain results in a subsequent metabolic alkalosis. Often hypokalaemia and hyponatraemia also ensues as the kidneys attempt to compensate.

Patients requiring long-term nasogastric suction include those in intensive care or as management for bowel obstruction. As with vomiting, there may be a metabolic alkalosis but in some cases there may be a metabolic acidosis due to loss of pancreatic secretions and bile (**Table 8.3**).

ABG measure	Level	Change
pH	7.51	↑
PCO_2 (kPa)	4.6	No change
PO_2 (kPa)	10.9	No change
HCO_3^- (mmol/L)	26.2	↑
Sodium (mmol/L)	138	No change
Potassium (mmol/L)	3.1	↓

Table 8.2 Arterial blood gases in significant vomiting.

ABG measure	Level	Change
pH	7.32	↓
PCO_2 (kPa)	4.8	No change
PO_2 (kPa)	11.2	No change
HCO_3^- (mmol/L)	19.2	↓
Sodium (mmol/L)	136	No change
Potassium (mmol/L)	3.0	↓

Table 8.3 Arterial blood gases in nasogastric suction.

8.3 Diarrhoea

Depending on the cause, diarrhoea can affect the acid–base balance of the blood in a number of complex ways. Severe, acute infective diarrhoea may cause a metabolic acidosis. This is because normal secretions into the gastrointestinal system are alkaline due to a high bicarbonate level. Up to 200 mL water is lost daily from plasma, and this leads to a normal anion gap acidosis (**Table 8.4**). If the diarrhoea is severe enough to cause hypovolaemia and shock, the resultant prerenal failure will contribute to the metabolic acidosis.

Diarrhoea that is not infective and affects the distal part of the gut can cause a metabolic alkalosis, due to the predominant loss of chloride into the gut. This is seen in diseases such as ulcerative colitis and typical ABGs are shown in **Table 8.5**. Finally, diarrhoea

ABG measure	Level	Change
pH	7.29	↓↓
PCO_2 (kPa)	3.8	↓
PO_2 (kPa)	15.2	↑
HCO_3^- (mmol/L)	18.2	↓
Sodium (mmol/L)	138	No change
Potassium (mmol/L)	3.2	↓

Table 8.4 Arterial blood gases in acute infective diarrhoea.

ABG measure	Level	Change
pH	7.49	↑
PCO_2 (kPa)	4.8	No change
PO_2 (kPa)	12.2	No change
HCO_3^- (mmol/L)	27.1	↑
Sodium (mmol/L)	140	No change
Potassium (mmol/L)	3.1	↓

Table 8.5 Arterial blood gases in distal gut diarrhoea.

associated with abdominal pain may lead to hyperventilation, resulting in a respiratory alkalosis as shown in **Table 8.6**.

8.4 Starvation

The acid–base mechanism in starvation (**Table 8.7**) is similar to that seen in diabetic ketoacidosis. Once the carbohydrate sources of energy are depleted, ketones and free fatty acids are used to provide energy.

Ketones in the urine may occur after just a few hours of starvation, but it takes several days for a metabolic acidosis to occur. Unlike the situation

> ### Clinical insight
>
> Starvation can be compounded in pregnancy: the mother may inherently become more dependent on fatty acid metabolism to allow the fetus to use glucose and carbohydrates.

ABG measure	Level	Change
pH	7.51	↑
PCO_2 (kPa)	2.9	↓↓
PO_2 (kPa)	17.1	↑↑
HCO_3^- (mmol/L)	20.2	No change
Sodium (mmol/L)	139	No change
Potassium (mmol/L)	4.8	No change

Table 8.6 Arterial blood gases in abdominal pain with hyperventilation.

ABG measure	Level	Change
pH	7.18	↓↓
PCO_2 (kPa)	2.8	↓↓
PO_2 (kPa)	17.9	↑↑
HCO_3^- (mmol/L)	14.1	↓↓
Sodium (mmol/L)	132	↓
Potassium (mmol/L)	5.6	↑
Glucose (mmol/L)	4.2	No change

Table 8.7 Arterial blood gases in starvation ketoacidosis.

in diabetic ketoacidosis, the relatively normal levels of insulin mean that there is often a rapid resolution of the metabolic acidosis with the intravenous administration of saline plus glucose or dextrose.

8.5 Diuretics

Use of thiazide and loop diuretics can cause a metabolic alkalosis (**Table 8.8**). This occurs due to increased sodium delivery to the distal tubules of the kidney. This also results in potassium loss because the increased sodium stimulates the aldosterone-sensitive sodium pump to increase sodium reabsorption, in exchange for potassium and hydrogen ions. These are excreted

ABG measure	Level	Change
pH	7.52	↑
PCO_2 (kPa)	4.2	No change
PO_2 (kPa)	10.8	No change
HCO_3^- (mmol/L)	27.2	↑
Sodium (mmol/L)	152	↑
Potassium (mmol/L)	2.9	↓↓

Table 8.8 Arterial blood gases in thiazide or loop diuretic usage

ABG measure	Level	Change
pH	7.29	↓↓
PCO_2 (kPa)	3.4	↓
PO_2 (kPa)	12.7	↑
HCO_3^- (mmol/L)	17.2	↓
Lactate	4.1	↑↑

Table 8.9 Arterial blood gases in cyanide poisoning.

into the urine and the resulting loss of hydrogen leads to metabolic alkalosis.

8.6 Cyanide poisoning

Cyanide poisoning can be deliberate, in cases of at-

> **Guiding principle**
>
> Potassium-sparing diuretics such as amiloride (a sodium channel blocker) and spironolactone (an aldosterone antagonist) can be used in conjunction with other diuretics to avoid hypokalaemia.

tempted murder or suicide, or accidental, in cases of smoke or chemical inhalation. The ABG may provide a useful clue prior to final diagnosis and typically shows a high anion gap, metabolic acidosis and a raised lactate, as shown in **Table 8.9**. The venous O_2 level may also be high (in some cases almost as high as the P_aCO_2), due to the inability of damaged cells to remove O_2 from the arterial blood.

Index

Note: Page numbers in **bold** or *italic* refer to tables or figures respectively.